Shunts

Congenitally corrected transpo c̄

VSD !

VSD
ASD
PDA
AP window → above A & v valve.   ductus
ruptured s.v aneurys   ...v or RA
coronary A-v fistula   , → RV, RA, PA
partial anom. venous.

Cyanosis c̄ ↑ vessels

Transpo (also DORV, Taussig Bing)
Truncus   Single vent c̄ PS
TAPVR   ─ Single vent !

↓ vessels

Tet & variants (Transpo c̄ PS)
                   (pseudotruncus, single vent c̄ PS
Ebsteins , Eisenmengers   DORV c̄ PS)
Tri Atresia
PS + PFO, ~~intact vent septum (looks the Ebstein)~~
~~Prisor of Fallot Trilogs~~
PA + intact septum - like Ebstein

Unequal flow - PS (↑ on Ⓛ)
              Tet (↓ on Ⓛ)(rt hypoplastic Ⓛ PA)
              Truncus - ↑ or ↓ anywhere
              Post Blalock

CARDIOVASCULAR RADIOLOGY

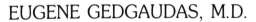

EUGENE GEDGAUDAS, M.D.

Professor and Chairman, Department of Radiology

JAMES H. MOLLER, M.D.

Professor of Pediatrics

WILFRIDO R. CASTANEDA-ZUNIGA, M.D.

Professor of Radiology

KURT AMPLATZ, M.D.

Professor of Radiology

University of Minnesota Medical School, Minneapolis, Minnesota

1985

W. B. SAUNDERS COMPANY

Philadelphia London Toronto Mexico City Rio de Janeiro Sydney Tokyo

W. B. Saunders Company: West Washington Square
Philadelphia, PA   19105

1 St. Anne's Road
Eastbourne, East Sussex BN21 3UN, England

1 Goldthorne Avenue
Toronto, Ontario M8Z 5T9, Canada

Apartado 26370—Cedro 512
Mexico 4, D.F., Mexico

Rua Coronel Cabrita, 8
Sao Cristovao Caixa Postal 21176
Rio de Janeiro, Brazil

9 Waltham Street
Artarmon, N.S.W. 2064, Australia

Ichibancho, Central Bldg., 22-1 Ichibancho
Chiyoda-Ku, Tokyo 102, Japan

Library of Congress Cataloging in Publication Data

Main entry under title:

Cardiovascular radiology.

1. Heart—Radiography.   2. Heart—Diseases—Diagnosis.
3. Heart—Abnormalities—Diagnosis.
4. Cardiovascular system—Diseases—Diagnosis.
5. Diagnosis, Radioscopic.   I. Gedgaudas, Eugene.
[DNLM: 1. Cardiovascular System—radiography.
WG 141.5.R2 C2675]

RC683.5.R3C37 1985   616.1′0757   84–10545

ISBN 0–7216–1084–6

Cardiovascular Radiology   ISBN 0-7216-1084-6

Last digit is the print number: 9   8   7   6   5   4   3   2   1

To all students and teachers
who have been associated with the
University of Minnesota
Variety Club Heart Hospital

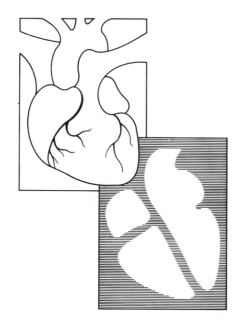

ACKNOWLEDGMENTS

We extend sincere thanks to our colleagues and associates at the University of Minnesota who helped to clarify our thinking about how to teach cardiovascular radiology. Dr. Richard G. Lester, now Dean and Vice President for Academic Affairs, Eastern Virginia Medical School, introduced E.G. and K.A. to the fascinating field of cardiovascular radiology. Dr. Jesse E. Edwards, Professor of Pathology, University of Minnesota, deserves special thanks for his superb teaching and continuing support in helping us to advance the science of cardiovascular radiology. Dr. Hugh Allen, Professor of Pediatrics, University of Arizona, helped greatly with our presentation of echocardiography. Dr. Zeev Vlodaver, Clinical Assistant Professor of Radiology, University of Minnesota, and Dr. Howard B. Burchell, Professor Emeritus, Cardiology, University of Minnesota, allowed us to share their expertise.

Thanks to Dr. Larry P. Elliott, Professor and Chairman of Radiology, Georgetown University, for keeping E.G.'s interest in cardiovascular radiology alive, and to Dr. Charles Higgins, Professor of Radiology, University of California, San Francisco, and Dr. Terry Ovitt, Professor of Radiology, University of Arizona, Tucson, for their case material incorporated in this book.

We also express our appreciation to Ms. Linda Richter, Medical Illustrator, Biomedical Graphics, University of Minnesota, for her outstanding work in creating the illustrations and for her helpful suggestions; Ms. Judith Bronson, for her editorial help; Ms. Linda Boche, for her meticulous care and aid in overall organization of the book; and Ms. Mary Jo Antinozzi, who helped in various ways in completion of this text.

E.G.
J.H.M.
W.R.C.-Z.
K.A.

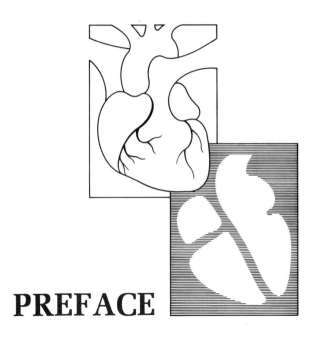

PREFACE

Clinical evaluation, an electrocardiogram, and roentgenographic examination of the chest with barium swallow form the classic triad of studies on which the diagnosis of cardiac disease rests. The four views of the heart recorded with barium in the esophagus give information about the state of the pulmonary vasculature, cardiac size and contour, any differential enlargement of the chambers, the relation and sizes of the great vessels, and the presence or absence of calcifications within the cardiac shadow or the vessels.

These roentgenographic findings may add new information or merely confirm the clinical impression. They may also have practical importance in planning a catheterization or surgical approach. For example, an aberrant right subclavian artery would preclude the use of the right brachial artery as an approach to the ascending aorta and left ventricle at cardiac catheterization. The discovery of a right aortic arch suggests to the surgeon a need to use the left subclavian artery for a Blalock-Taussig anastomosis.

Most congenital and acquired cardiac conditions can be diagnosed with reasonable accuracy using basic radiologic skills, although clinical information always increases the likelihood of accurate diagnosis. This is particularly true in congenital heart disease. Such information as the presence or absence of cyanosis, the presence of significant murmurs, or electrocardiographic findings is of paramount importance in reaching a definitive diagnosis.

Since the American Board of Radiology established a special examination in cardiovascular radiology in 1979, the need for structured teaching of the subject has become apparent. Our purpose has been to provide, in an attractive and readable format, the essential information that the radiologist needs to understand cardiovascular radiology. By adopting a systematic physiologic approach with emphasis on plain film diagnosis, we aim to improve the reader's ability to use

v

roentgenographic findings to determine whether the heart is normal or not and to place each abnormality in the appropriate physiologic group. To this end, anatomic, hemodynamic and clinical background material is employed to assist the reader in understanding the radiographic abnormalities.

EUGENE GEDGAUDAS, M.D.
JAMES H. MOLLER, M.D.
WILFRIDO R. CASTANEDA-ZUNIGA, M.D.
KURT AMPLATZ, M.D.

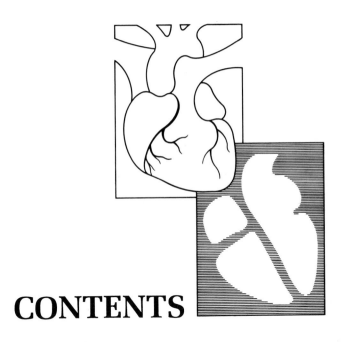

CONTENTS

THE CENTRAL CIRCULATION IN CONGENITAL HEART DISEASE

(Page numbers refer to discussions in the text)

Ao	Aorta
LA	Left atrium
LV	Left ventricle
PA	Pulmonary artery
RA	Right atrium
RV	Right ventricle
ACPV	Anomalous connecting pulmonary vein
SVC	Superior vena cava
Port V	Portal vein

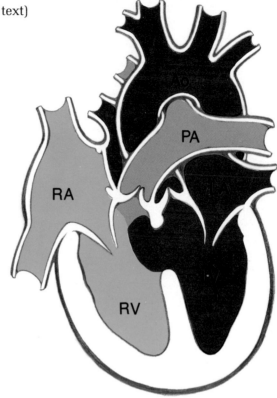

Large ventricular septal defect (p. 68)

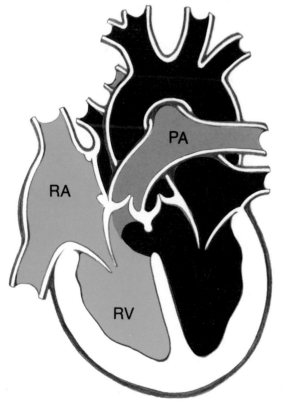

Small ventricular septal defect (p. 68)

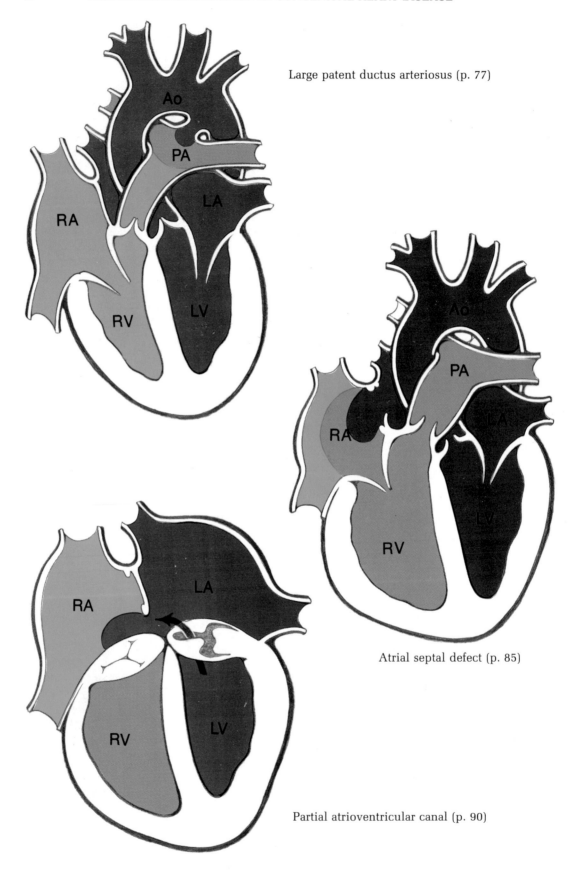

Large patent ductus arteriosus (p. 77)

Atrial septal defect (p. 85)

Partial atrioventricular canal (p. 90)

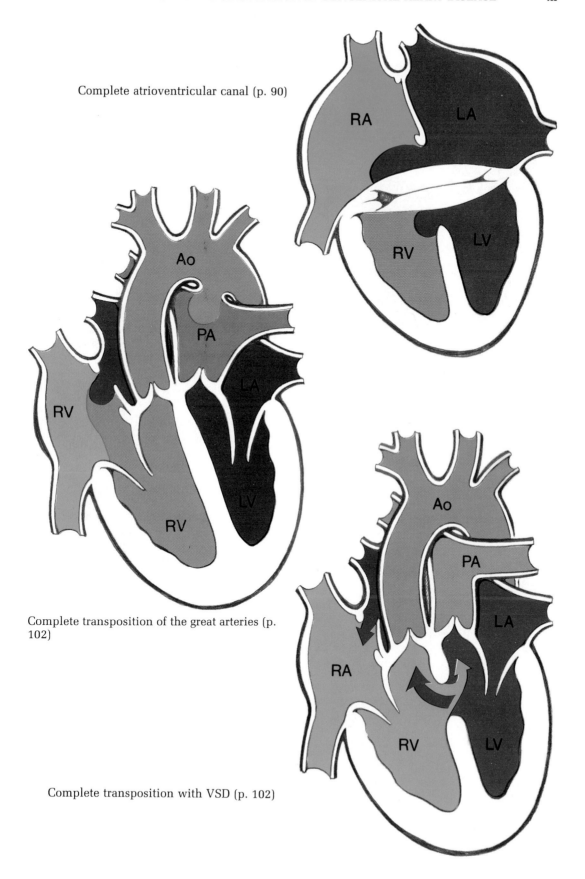

Complete atrioventricular canal (p. 90)

Complete transposition of the great arteries (p. 102)

Complete transposition with VSD (p. 102)

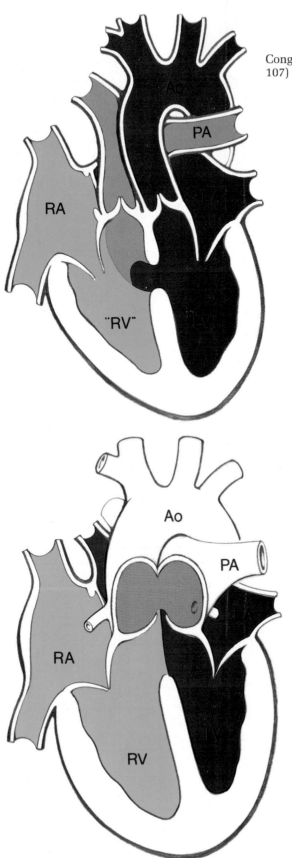

Congenitally corrected transposition with VSD (p. 107)

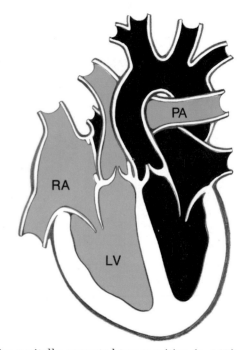

Congenitally corrected transposition (p. 107)

Persistent truncus arteriosus (p. 112)

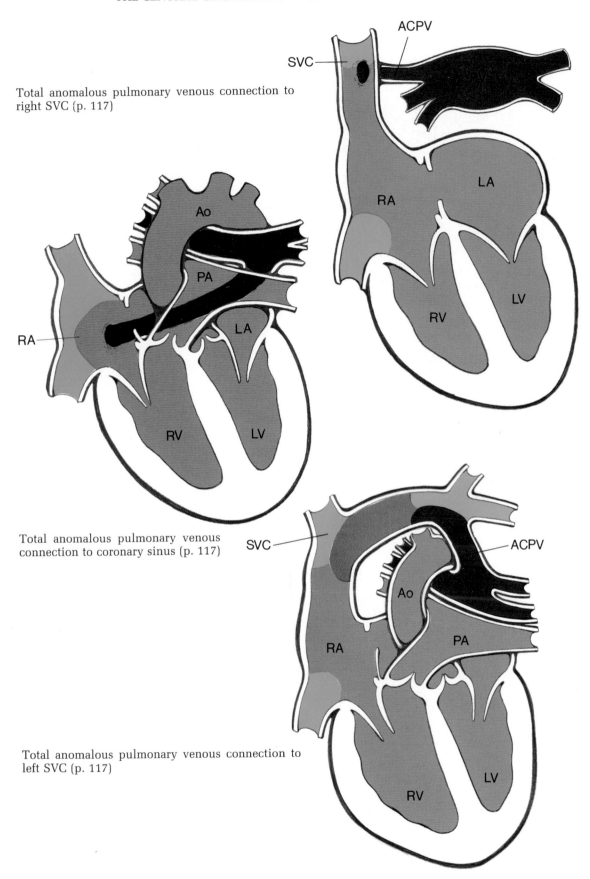

Total anomalous pulmonary venous connection to right SVC (p. 117)

Total anomalous pulmonary venous connection to coronary sinus (p. 117)

Total anomalous pulmonary venous connection to left SVC (p. 117)

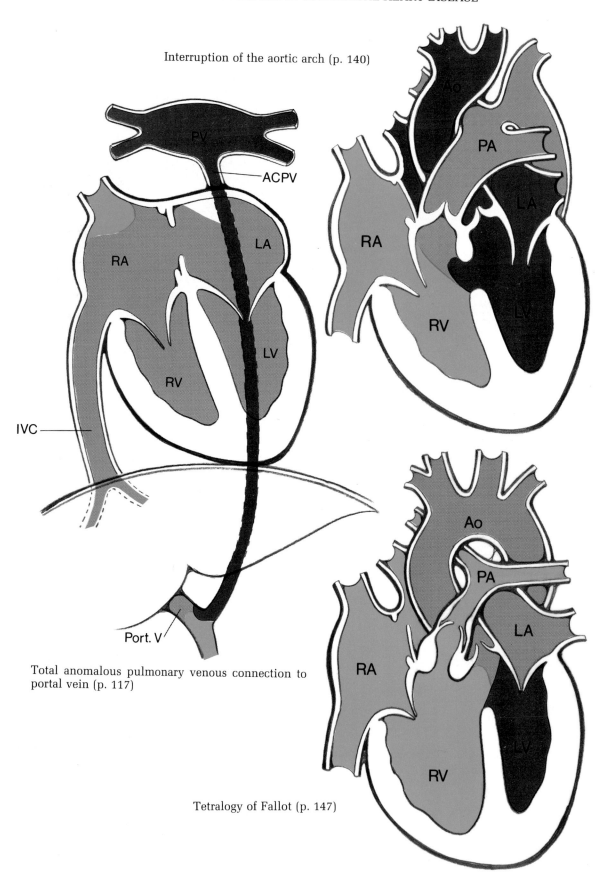

Interruption of the aortic arch (p. 140)

Total anomalous pulmonary venous connection to portal vein (p. 117)

Tetralogy of Fallot (p. 147)

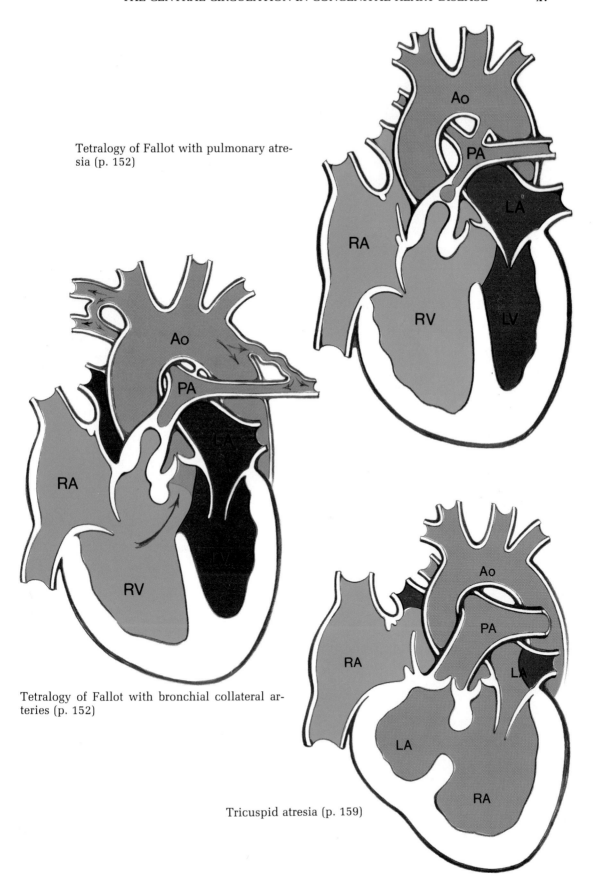

Tetralogy of Fallot with pulmonary atresia (p. 152)

Tetralogy of Fallot with bronchial collateral arteries (p. 152)

Tricuspid atresia (p. 159)

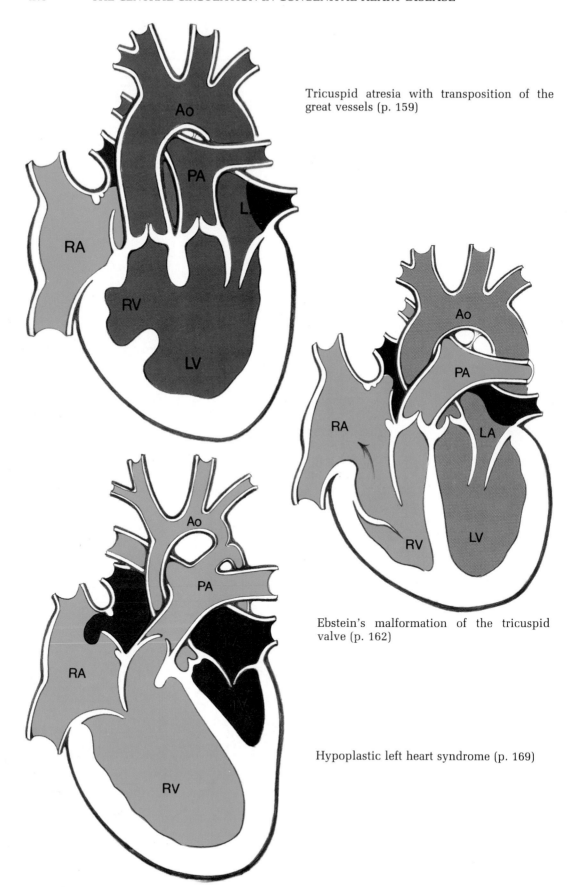

Tricuspid atresia with transposition of the great vessels (p. 159)

Ebstein's malformation of the tricuspid valve (p. 162)

Hypoplastic left heart syndrome (p. 169)

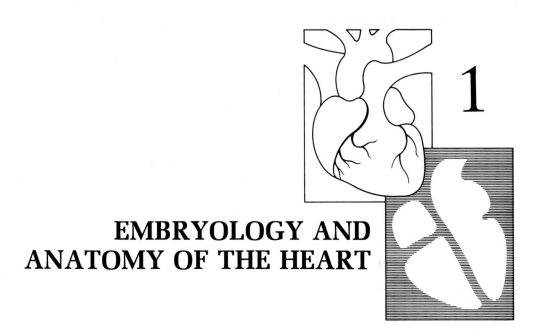

EMBRYOLOGY AND ANATOMY OF THE HEART

EMBRYOLOGY

To help in understanding the anatomic details of congenital cardiac malfor-mations, this brief review of normal cardiac embryology is presented.

After 18 days of embryonic development, two cardiac cords form which then become canalized to form endothelial tubes; by 21 days these begin to fuse into a single cardiac tube beginning at the cranial end. The cardiac tube elongates, and external constrictions mark its several segments: *the sinus venosus,* which receives the umbilical, vitelline, and common cardinal veins; *atrium; ventricularis; bulbus cordis; truncus arteriosus; aortic sac;* and *aortic arches* (Fig. 1–1). Because the cardiac tube is fixed and attached at the sinus venosus and arterial ends, it bends upon itself as it elongates, forming an **S**. Initially, the **S**-shaped bulboventricular

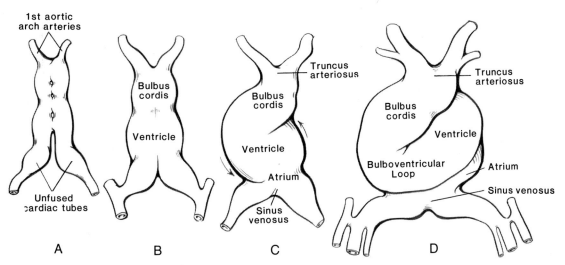

FIGURE 1–1. Embryologic development of the cardiac tube. *A,* Paired cardiac tubes fuse in cephalad to caudad direction. *B,* Fused cadiac tube with beginning chamber differentiation. *C,* Beginning rotation of cardiac tube to right. *D,* Further rotation of cardiac tube to right. Various segments of heart well delineated.

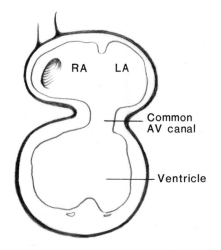

FIGURE 1–2. Embryologic development of the atrioventricular canal. Cross-section through common atrium (above) and common ventricle (below). The atrioventricular canal, at this stage, connects the left side of the atrium to the left side of the common ventricle.

loop is directed toward the the right, and the atrium and sinus venosus move posteriorly behind the ventricle.

The primitive atrium and ventricle communicate through the atrioventricular canal, which gradually shifts toward the right, so that it lies above the developing left and right ventricles and beneath the left and right atria (Fig. 1–2). The atrioventricular canal is then divided by the developing endocardial cushions, one of which arises dorsally and the other ventrally. The endocardial cushions fuse, dividing the common atrioventricular canal into separate canals, one connecting the right atrium and right ventricle and the other the left atrium and left ventricle (Fig. 1–3).

The primitive atrium is partitioned by a series of events (Fig. 1–4). A thin, crescent-shaped membrane, the *septum primum,* develops along the cranial wall of the atrium and grows caudally toward the fused endocardial cushions. The space between the advancing margin of the septum primum and the endocardial cushion is called the *ostium primum,* and this gradually shrinks, disappearing when the free edge of the septum primum fuses completely with the left side of the endocardial cushions. However, before this fusion occurs, perforations form in the septum primum and coalesce to form the *ostium secundum.* A second crescent-shaped membrane forms on the ventral and cranial wall of the atrium immediately to the right of the septum primum and gradually grows toward the endocardial cushions, covering the ostium secundum. It does not reach the endocardial cushions, and its crescent-shaped lower margin forms the foramen ovale.

The primitive ventricle is also divided by a series of events (Fig. 1–3). First, an interventricular septum with a crescentic upper edge forms, and the ventricles expand and dilate on either side of this septum. Subsequently, there is active growth of the muscular septum toward the endocardial cushions. The space above the developing interventricular septum and the endocardial cushions is called the *interventricular foramen.* Its closure occurs by the fusion of endocardial cushion tissue with the bulbar ventricular ridges, which, after dividing the primitive truncus, extend into the ventricle.

The truncus arteriosus and bulbus cordis are divided by paired ridges of subendocardial tissue—bulbar ridges—which eventually fuse in the midline, forming the aorticopulmonary septum. The spiral-shaped septum divides the truncus arteriosus into two channels, the aorta and the pulmonary artery (Fig. 1–5). The bulbar ridges also cross the bulbar ventricular region and contribute to the

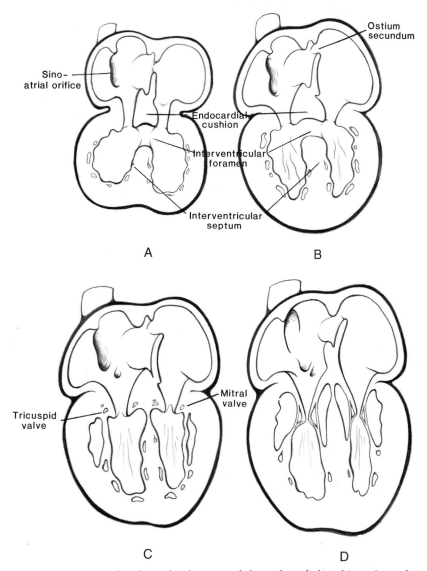

FIGURE 1–3. Embryologic development of the endocardial cushions. Later development stage. Anteroposterior view. *A,* Endocardial cushion tissue has developed and split the common atrioventricular canal. *B,* Atrial communication—ostium secundum (above)—and ventricular septal defect (below). Endocardial cushion tissue continues to develop and differentiate. *C,* Endocardial cushion has sealed, closing the ventricular septum. Endocardial cushion beginning to differentiate into valvular tissue. *D,* Complete differentiation by endocardial cushion tissue into septae and the septal leaflets of the tricuspid and mitral valves.

formation of the upper portion of the ventricular septum and of the semilunar cusps; three of these cusps are formed in each great artery from the ridges and the dorsal and ventral endocardial cushions at the bulbar ventricular junction.

Early in embryonic development the venous system is bilateral and symmetrical, and the two sides empty into the left and right horns of the sinus venosus (Fig. 1–6). Gradually, the left-sided venous system—principally the left anterior and posterior cardinal veins—regresses, and eventually, the only major remnant is a portion of the coronary sinus. Simultaneously the left horn of the sinus venosus regresses and the right horn expands as it receives the entire systemic

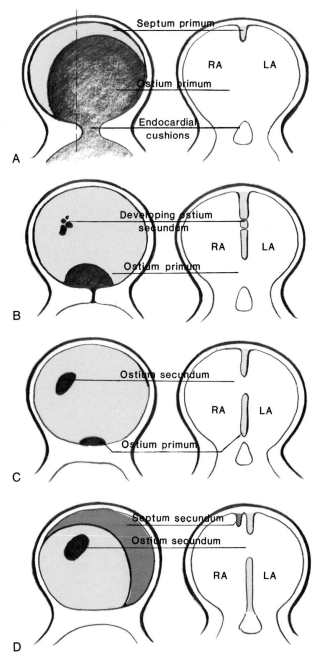

FIGURE 1–4. Development of the interatrial septum. Right lateral and anterior views. The septum primum is shown in dark gray and the septum secundum in light gray. *A,* Beginning development of the ostium primum and septum primum. The large communication between the atria is the ostium primum. *B,* Progressive development of the septum primum. Reduction in size of the ostium primum. Perforations forming in the septum primum. *C,* Further reduction in size of the ostium primum due to growth of the septum primum. Coalescence of perforations forms the ostium secundum. *D,* Septum primum fused with endocardial cushions, enlargement of the ostium secundum, and initial development of the septum secundum in the right atrium.

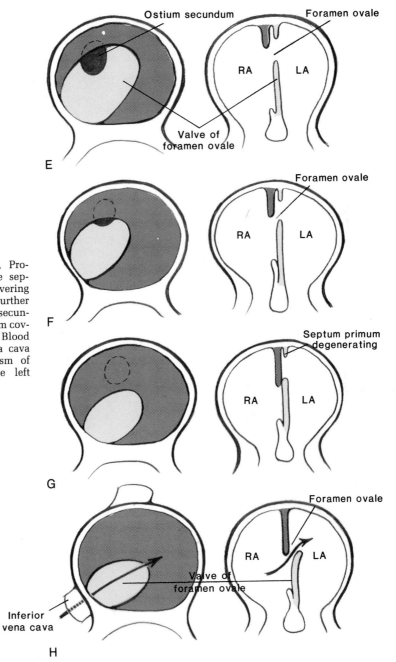

FIGURE 1–4 *Continued. E, Progressive development of the septum secundum, partially covering the ostium secundum. F, Further development of the septum secundum. G, The septum secundum covers the ostium secundum. H, Blood flows from the inferior vena cava through flap-valve mechanism of the atrial septum into the left atrium.*

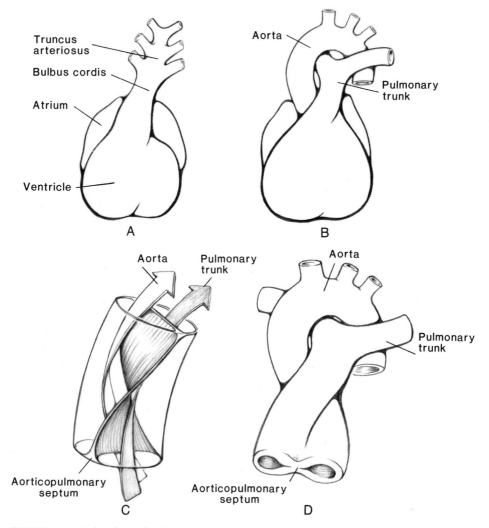

FIGURE 1–5. Embryologic development of the great arteries. *A*, A common vessel, the truncus arteriosus, originates from the primitive ventricular loop, giving rise to paired aortic arches. *B*, Separation of the great arteries. *C*, Intertwining of the two great arteries as they leave the heart. *D*, Separation of the truncus arteriosus by ingrowth of a spiral septum which develops cephalad to caudad. In this illustration separation is incomplete.

venous return through the inferior and superior venae cavae. The right horn of the sinus venosus becomes incorporated into the posterior wall of the right atrium.

Initially, the pulmonary venous system is connected to the systemic venous system, but gradually, individual pulmonary veins differentiate within the lungs and form a confluence behind the region of the left atrium (Fig. 1–7). From the left atrium, a projection, the common pulmonary vein, extends to join this confluence. This communication then expands, and the connection with the systemic veins regresses and eventually disappears. The communication between the left atrium and pulmonary veins continues to enlarge, until the confluence forms the posterior wall of the left atrium with the pulmonary veins entering individually.

The truncus arteriosus ends in the aortic sac and, from the latter, symmetrical aortic arches arise which extend dorsally to the paired dorsal aortae. Eventually,

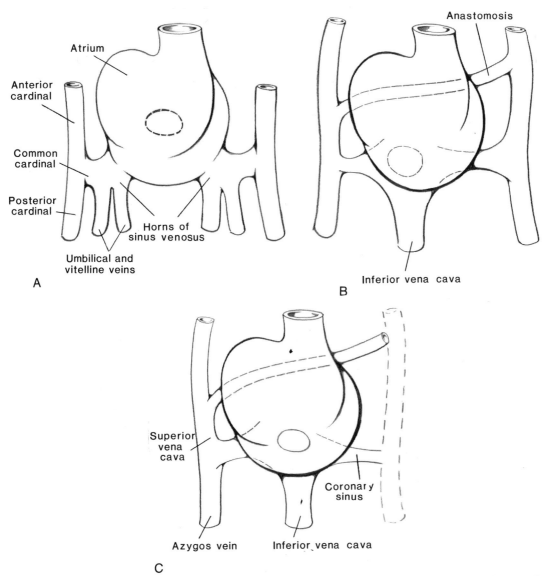

FIGURE 1–6. Development of the systemic venous system. *A,* Bilateral anterior cardinal and posterior cardinal join common cardinal vein. Umbilical and vitelline veins join common cardinal and form horns of sinus venosus to join atrium. *B,* Anastomosis develops between left and right anterior cardinals. Changes have taken place in inferior vena cava. *C,* Remnants of left cardinal system have disappeared except for coronary sinus. The anastomotic vessel (remnant of right anterior cardinal) enlarges and joins the superior vena cava.

six paired aortic arches develop, although not all are present at any one time (Fig. 1–8). Portions of these arches regress and disappear; the remnants are:

Arch I. Part of the maxillary arteries
Arch II. Part of the stapedial arteries
Arch III. The common carotid arteries
Arch IV. The aortic arch and part of the right subclavian artery
Arch V. No derivatives

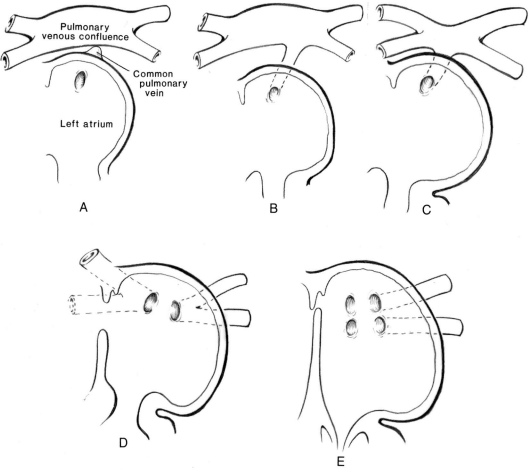

FIGURE 1–7. Incorporation of the pulmonary veins into the left atrium. *A,* Confluence of the pulmonary veins has formed. From the left atrium a projection (the common pulmonary vein) develops. *B,* The common pulmonary vein makes contact with the confluence of the pulmonary veins. *C,* The opening between the left atrium and the confluence broadens. *D,* Broader opening between the confluence and the pulmonary veins. *E,* Final incorporation of the confluence into the left atrium with separate opening of each pulmonary vein.

> Arch VI. The proximal part of the left pulmonary artery and distal part of the ductus arteriosus (left), and the proximal part of the right pulmonary artery (right). (The distal part usually disappears. If present, it represents a right patent ductus arteriosus.)

Early in embryonic development, the two dorsal aortae begin to fuse in the abdomen, with the fusion progressing toward the thorax. The right dorsal aorta in the thorax gradually regresses, leaving only the left dorsal aorta as the descending thoracic aorta.

The Fetal Circulation

The fetal circulation has four unique anatomic structures—the placenta, the ductus venosus, the foramen ovale, and the ductus arteriosus—that are integral during fetal life but disappear after birth. Knowledge of the fetal circulatory system helps one understand both the natural history of certain congenital cardiac malformations and the circulatory changes that may occur in sick neonates, particularly those with pulmonary disease.

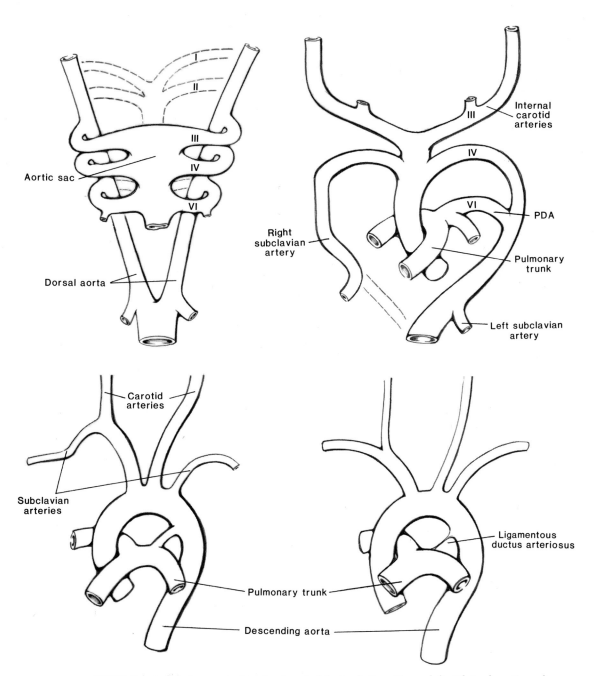

FIGURE 1–8. Development of systemic arterial circulation. *Upper left,* Bilateral aortic arches leave aortic sac and pass posteriorly into dorsal aorta. The first (I) and second (II) arches have involuted. *Upper right,* Further progression in development. The branches of the third (III) arch form the internal carotid arteries. The left fourth (IV) aortic arch persists as the aortic arch and the sixth (VI) persists as the ductus arteriosus. The proximal right fourth (IV) arch and a portion of the right dorsal aorta form the right subclavian artery. *Lower left,* Migration of subclavian arteries has occurred so that they are more proximal on the arch. *Lower right,* Following birth, normal patterns of the aortic arch and pulmonary trunk persist. Ligamentous ductus arteriosus remains as the only remnant of the sixth (VI) arch.

Fetal Circulation

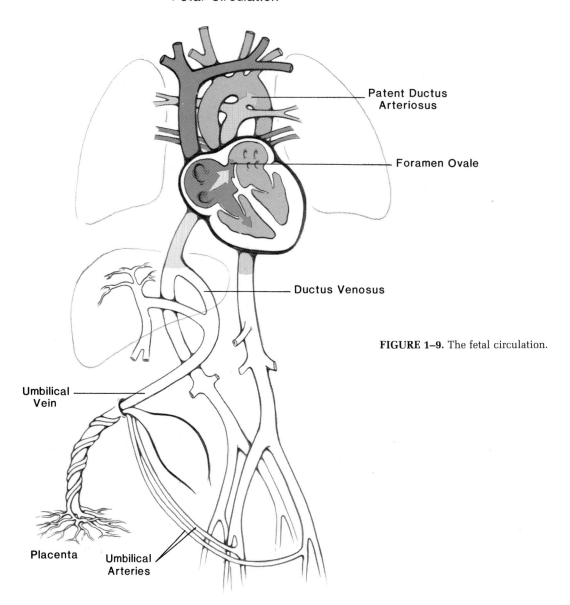

Patent Ductus Arteriosus

Foramen Ovale

Ductus Venosus

Umbilical Vein

Placenta

Umbilical Arteries

FIGURE 1–9. The fetal circulation.

The placenta is the principal site of oxygenation and metabolic exchange for the fetus and receives 40 per cent of the fetal cardiac output. The oxygenated blood from the placenta returns via the umbilical veins; most of it bypasses the liver through the ductus venosus to enter the inferior vena cava (Fig. 1–9), while a small amount passes through the portal system to enter the right lobe of the liver. The inferior vena caval blood reaches the right atrium. It is directed by the lower margin of the septum secundum, the *crista dividens,* through the foramen ovale into the left atrium, where it mixes with a small amount of unoxygenated blood returning from the pulmonary veins. The left atrial blood passes into the left ventricle and through the ascending aorta, supplying the brain predominantly.

TABLE 1–1. DISTRIBUTION OF BLOOD FLOW IN FETUS*

SITE	FLOW (%)	SATURATION (%)
Right ventricle	66	55
Ductus	59	55
Pulmonary artery	7	55
Descending aorta	69	60
Left ventricle	34	65
Aortic isthmus	10	65
Inferior vena cava	69	70
Superior vena cava	21	40
Foramen ovale	27	–
Placenta	40–50	–

*Flow expressed in percentage of combined left and right ventricular outputs; percentage of oxygen saturation from various sites given.

Only a small volume of the left ventricular output crosses the aortic isthmus to enter the descending aorta. The blood returning to the heart through the superior vena cava passes preferentially into the right ventricle and then into the pulmonary trunk.

Because the resistance to blood flow through the fetal lung is high, particularly in comparison with the systemic resistance (which is lowered by the spacious vascular bed of the placenta), little blood flows through the lungs. The principal blood flow from the pulmonary trunk occurs from right to left through the ductus arteriosus into the descending aorta. Most blood in the descending aorta is delivered either to the placenta or to the kidneys. Representative oxygen saturations and volumes of blood flow are given in Table 1–1.

The fetal circulation is one in which the systemic and pulmonary circulations function in parallel, with the volume of blood flowing into each circuit being determined principally by the systemic and pulmonary vascular resistances. After birth, profound anatomic and hemodynamic changes occur (Fig. 1–10). The elimination of the placenta from the circulation causes an immediate increase in systemic vascular resistance and a cessation of blood return through the umbilical vein and ductus venosus; the latter structure becomes obliterated between the third and seventh days of life.

The other major change occurs with the expansion of the lungs. Pulmonary vascular resistance decreases significantly, principally because the improved oxygenation lessens the hypoxic pulmonary vasoconstriction. As a result, pulmonary blood flow increases markedly. The greatly increased volume of blood returning to the left atrium raises the left atrial pressure and functionally closes the foramen ovale within minutes of birth. During the first year of life, the foramen ovale becomes anatomically sealed in 75 per cent of individuals.

During the first six hours of life, a bidirectional flow occurs through the ductus arteriosus. As pulmonary vascular resistance and pulmonary arterial pressure fall, the flow becomes left to right. In full-term infants, constriction of the media of the ductus arteriosus causes functional closure by 24 hours of age, and anatomic closure generally occurs by 10 days of age, beginning at the pulmonary arterial end and progressing toward the aorta. The factors causing ductal closure have not been fully identified. Increased oxygen concentration is known to be a potent ductal constrictor, whereas hypoxemia tends to open the ductus in neonates.

Neonatal Circulation

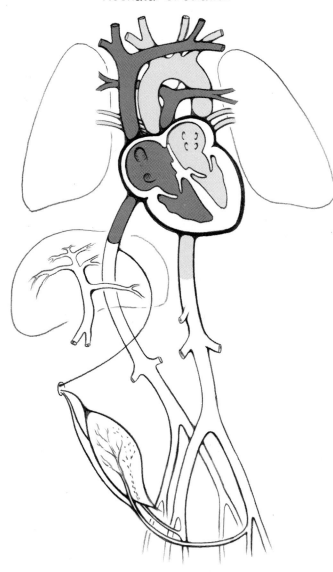

FIGURE 1–10. The neonatal circulation.

Selected Bibliography

de la Cruz, M. V., Gomez, C. S., Arteaga, M. M., and Arguello, C.: Experimental study of the development of the truncus and the conus in the chick embryo. J. Anat. *123*:661–686, 1977.

Dische, M. R.: Observations on the morphological changes of the developing heart. Pediatr. Cardiol. 2:176–191, 1980.

CARDIAC ANATOMY

The heart lies predominately in the left hemithorax immediately behind the sternum. The interatrial and interventricular septae lie in a vertical plane that is directed toward the left midclavicular line and intersects the anterior chest wall at a 45 degree angle to the midline. Therefore, the right atrium and ventricle are located anteriorly to the left atrium and ventricle. When the heart is seen from the front, its right border is formed by the right atrium, while its left border is composed of the aortic knob, pulmonary trunk, left atrial appendage, and left ventricle. In addition, the ouflow area of the right ventricle directly overlies, and wraps partly around, the outflow area of the left ventricle so that the two outflow tracts cross nearly at a right angle, with the right ventricular area being directed superiorly to the left and the left ventricular area being directed superiorly to the right. Cognizance of this relationship is essential for interpreting thoracic roentgenograms and angiocardiograms.

Right Atrium

The free wall of the right atrium consists of two parts: a smooth-walled posterior part, which is derived from the embryonic sinus venosus; and a thin-walled trabeculated part, composing the embryonic right atrium. The two portions are separated by a muscular ridge, the *crista terminalis,* which is most prominent superiorly near the orifice of the superior vena cava and fades out to the right of the orifice of the inferior vena cava. This ridge corresponds to the external *sulcus terminalis.* Several parallel pectinate muscles pass laterally and anteriorly from the crista terminalis; between them, the atrial wall is thin and translucent. These muscles extend into the triangular right atrial appendage, which is located anteriorly and superiorly.

The medial wall of the right atrium is the atrial septum which is smooth except for a central depressed area, the *fossa ovalis.* The elevated thickened margin of this area is called the *limbus of the fossa ovalis.*

Systemic venous blood returns to the heart through the superior and inferior venae cavae and the coronary sinus and enters the smooth portion of the right atrium. The superior vena caval orifice opens freely, whereas the orifice of the inferior vena cava, which partly faces the fossa ovalis, may be guarded by the *eustachian valve.* The size of this valve, which is attached along the crista terminalis, is variable; in some persons, the valve is absent. In others, the valve is perforated *(network of Chiari).* The coronary sinus enters anteriorly and medially to the inferior vena caval orifice; it, too, may be guarded by a small flap of tissue, the *thebesian valve.* Both the eustachian and thebesian valves derive from the embryonic right sinus venosus valve.

Right Ventricle

The tricuspid valve is located anteromedially and connects the chamber of the right atrium with that of the right ventricle. Its three leaflets—anterior, medial (septal), and posterior—are opened by two distinct papillary muscles, a smaller medial muscle attached by chordae tendineae to the anterior and medial leaflets, and a larger anterior muscle attached to the anterior and posterior leaflets. The posterior leaflet is also tethered by numerous small papillary muscles along the diaphragmatic portion of the right ventricle.

The ventricle is divided into two portions, a posteroinferior (inflow or sinus) portion and an anterosuperior (outflow or conus) portion, which lie roughly at right angles to one another. The sinus portion is heavily trabeculated, particularly in the apical region, with muscle fascicles called *trabeculae carneae.* The conus portion is less trabeculated and gives rise to the medial papillary muscle. The subpulmonary region of the conus is smooth.

The sinus and conus portions of the ventricle are separated by the *crista supraventricularis,* a well-developed muscular ridge that lies posteriorly. The ridge is composed of two bands—the parietal, which extends onto the free wall of the ventricle, and the septal, which extends onto the interventricular septum. A portion of the septal band, called the moderator band, gives rise to the anterior papillary muscle and contains the right *bundle of His.*

A small portion of the membranous intraventricular septum is located beneath the medial leaflet of the tricuspid valve. A large portion lies above the tricuspid annulus.

Pulmonary Circulation

The semilunar *pulmonary valve,* which has three cusps, lies between the right ventricle and the pulmonary trunk, which passes superiorly, posteriorly, and slightly to the left before dividing into the left and right pulmonary arteries.

The left pulmonary artery appears as a direct extension of the pulmonary trunk and arches dorsally to the left. As it passes into the left pulmonary hilus, it courses over and behind the left mainstem bronchus. The *ligamentum arteriosum* arises from the superior surface of the proximal portion of the left pulmonary artery.

The right pulmonary artery arises at a right angle from the pulmonary trunk and passes behind the ascending aorta. It lies in front of the right mainstem bronchus.

Normally, two pairs of pulmonary veins return blood to the left atrium. The left superior and inferior veins enter the left lateral posterior part of the chamber. The right superior vein passes behind the superior vena cava, and the right inferior vein passes behind the smooth portion of the right atrium. The two right-sided veins then enter the posteromedial portion of the left atrium near the atrial septum.

Left Atrium

The left atrium is the most posterior of the cardiac chambers and lies in the midline below the carina of the trachea and the mainstem bronchi. Posteriorly, it touches the esophagus. Its transverse diameter is greater than either its vertical or its anteroposterior diameter, and its wall is smooth and thick. The left atrial appendage contains fewer pectinate muscles and is longer and narrower than the right atrial appendage.

The surface of the interatrial septum is smoother in the left atrium than in the right. The valve of the foramen ovale overlies the area of the fossa ovalis. Its inferior margin, a remnant of the septum primum, may be scalloped.

Left Ventricle

Blood flows anteriorly to the left through the left atrium and *mitral valve* into the left ventricle, which comprises most of the posterior and left lateral aspect of the heart and is in contact with the esophagus.

The two leaflets of the mitral valve are attached to the atrioventricular annulus. The larger, anterior (septal) leaflet lies opposite the interventricular septum and extends to the posterior (noncoronary) aortic cusp. The smaller and more variably sized posterior leaflet lies along the left aspect of the ventricle. Two papillary muscles, the anterolateral and posteromedial, project into the ventricle; their chordae tendineae insert into each leaflet.

The conical, thick-walled left ventricle is separated into an inflow portion, posterior to the anterior leaflet of the mitral valve, and an anterior outflow portion. The translucent membranous interventricular septum is located in the angle between the right and posterior cusps of the aortic valve.

Systemic Arterial Circulation

The aortic valve guards the passage from the left ventricle to the aorta. It is a semilunar valve with three leaflets: posterior (noncoronary), right, and left. The leaflets are thin and pocket-like and, when closed, they form the sinuses of Valsalva. Above this level, the coronary arteries arise—the left artery above the left cusp and the right and conal branches above the right cusp. The aorta forms a gentle arch, passing superiorly, then dorsally and slightly to the left, and finally posteriorly. From its arch arise three major arteries—the innominate, the left carotid, and the left subclavian.

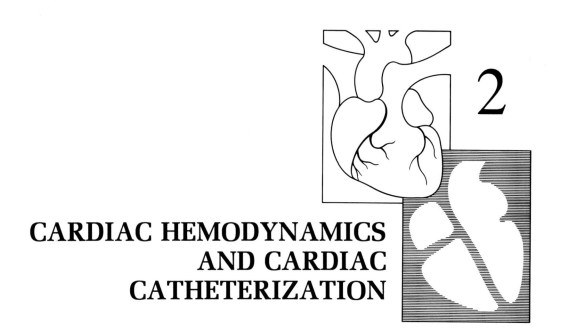

CARDIAC HEMODYNAMICS AND CARDIAC CATHETERIZATION

THE CARDIAC CYCLE

To understand the hemodynamics of various cardiac anomalies and conditions, it is helpful to review the events and relations that occur during the cardiac cycle.

The sequential depolarization of the atrium and ventricle is indicated on the electrocardiogram by the P wave and QRS complex, respectively (Fig. 2–1). Coincident with the QRS complex, the ventricles begin to contract, and simultaneous contraction of the papillary muscles closes the mitral and tricuspid valves. The closure of these atrioventricular valves marks the beginning of the isovolumetric contraction period, a short phase of the cardiac cycle during which all of the cardiac valves are closed, the intraventricular pressure begins to rise, and no blood is moving within the heart. As the ventricles continue to contract, the pressure increases until it reaches and then exceeds the pressure in the great arteries, thus opening the aortic and pulmonary valves. The opening of these valves marks the end of the isovolumetric contraction and the beginning of the systolic ejection phase, during which each ventricle is in communication with its corresponding great artery, the systolic pressure continues to rise, and blood is ejected. Pressures reach a peak during the middle of the ejection phase and then, as the volume of ejection begins to decrease, the systolic pressure begins to fall. Systolic ejection ends when the pressure in the ventricle falls below that of the corresponding great artery. At that precise point, the ejection phase ends, the semilunar valves close, and the period of isovolumetric relaxation begins. During this brief period, all cardiac valves are again closed, the ventricular pressure is falling, and no blood is flowing within the heart. In the great arteries, the pressure remains elevated, in part because of the closed similunar valves.

The ventricular pressure continues to decline and, when it falls below the pressure of the corresponding atrium, the atrioventricular valves open. The opening marks the end of the isovolumetric relaxation period and the beginning of the rapid ventricular filling phase of diastole. Approximately 60 per cent of the blood flow into a ventricle occurs in the first 20 per cent of diastole. After this rapid filling phase, the slow filling phase occurs, occupying the mid part of diastole

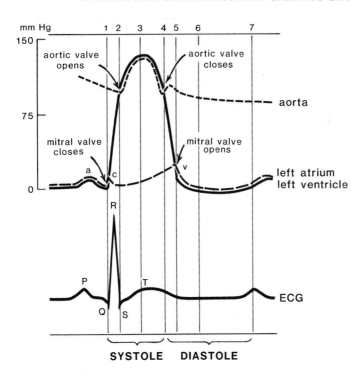

FIGURE 2–1. Relationship between the electrocardiogram (ECG) and the cardiac cycle. Changes of normal left atrial, left ventricular, and aortic pressure throughout the cardiac cycle are shown. Periods of the cardiac cycle: *1–2,* isovolumetric contraction; *2–3,* ejection phase to peak systolic pressure; *3–4,* systolic ejection phase to dicrotic notch occurring at site 4; *4–5,* period of isovolumetric relaxation; *5–6,* rapid ventricular filling phase; *6–7,* slow ventricular filling phase. The left atrial pressure curve has three distinct wave forms: *a,* atrial contraction, *c,* occurring during isovolumetric contraction, and *v,* reaching a peak at opening of the mitral valve. ECG wave forms: *P,* atrial depolarization, *QRS,* ventricular depolarization, *T,* ventricular repolarization.

with another 20 per cent of ventricular filling. The last phase of diastole, corresponding with atrial contraction, occurs with the P wave of the electrocardiogram in which the final 20 per cent of ventricular filling occurs. Throughout diastole, the atrial pressure is slightly higher than that in the corresponding ventricle. Ventricular repolarization, represented by the T wave of the electrocardiogram, occurs during diastole but does not influence any of the hemodynamic events.

Various heart sounds can be heard during the cardiac cycle, most of which mark the transition between phases (Fig. 2–1). The principal normal and abnormal heart sounds are:

S_1 = First heart sound, corresponding to the closure of the atrioventricular valves and the beginning of isovolumetric contraction

SEC = Systolic ejection click, corresponding to the opening of the semilunar valves and the end of isovolumetric contraction; an *abnormal sound*, indicating dilatation of a great vessel

S_2 = Second heart sound, corresponding to the closure of the semilunar valves and the end of the ejection phase

OS = Opening snap, corresponding to the opening of the atrioventricular valve and the end of isovolumetric relaxation; an *abnormal sound*, indicating stenosis

S_3 = Third heart sound, marking the transition between the rapid and slow filling phase

S_4 = Fourth heart sound, occurring with atrial contraction; normal in older adults but *abnormal* in children

CARDIAC CATHETERIZATION

Cardiac catheterization is performed to establish a diagnosis, assess the severity of an abnormality, or evaluate the effect of a cardiac condition on the heart and circulation. These can be accomplished by several means:

1. Observing the course of the catheter

2. Measuring the pressures in the cardiac chambers and great vessels
3. Measuring oxygen content of the chambers and great vessels (oximetry)
4. Performing angiography
5. Performing specialized tests, e.g., dye curves

These measurements may be made with the patient at rest. Often, however, it is important to know the response of the heart to stress. With these patients, a bicycle ergometer may be attached to the front of the catheterization table and the patient asked to pedal the bicycle against resistance. After a steady exercise state has been reached, pressure measurements and oximetric data may be obtained. Measurements of blood flow and intracardiac pressure may also be made during and after the administration of cardioactive drugs.

Catheter Course

The normal course of the catheter is easily recognizable by fluoroscopy. The course is abnormal in patients with abnormal internal or external communications such as ventricular septal defect or patent ductus arteriosus, or with abnormalities in the course of the major veins and arteries (Fig. 2–2). For instance, if a catheter passes from one ventricle to the other, this is strong evidence of a ventricular septal defect.

Pressure Measurements

During cardiac catheterization, pressures are measured in each cardiac chamber and great vessel that the catheter enters. A pulmonary capillary, or wedge, pressure is usually measured by advancing the tip of an end-hole catheter as far as possible into the lung field and wedging it into the pulmonary artery. The catheter prevents the forward transmission of the pulmonary arterial pressure; therefore, the pressure measured at this site reflects that in the pulmonary capillary bed, which, in most people, is the same as the pulmonary venous and left atrial pressures. Measurements of intracardiac pressures are used (1) to establish a diagnosis—for instance, in valvular stenosis, in which a pressure gradient can be measured across a valve; (2) to assess the severity of the condition—for instance, determining the degree of pulmonary hypertension in a patient with a ventricular septal defect; and (3) to assess the effect of a malformation on myocardial function—for instance, measuring ventricular end-diastolic pressure or the pressure changes caused by exercise.

The right atrial pressure is normally 2 to 5 mm Hg. An elevated pressure usually means right ventricular failure, reduced right ventricular compliance, or the rare conditions, tricuspid stenosis or insufficiency.

The right ventricular pressure is normally 25/0 to 5 mm Hg. Systolic pressure becomes elevated through pulmonary hypertension or by conditions such as transposition of the great vessels or truncus arteriosus, in which the right ventricle is connected to the systemic circulation, or when there is some form of pulmonary stenosis. In the latter instance, a systolic gradient is found between the pulmonary artery and the right ventricle. The right ventricular diastolic pressure is elevated in the presence of right ventricular failure, reduced right ventricular compliance because of ventricular hypertrophy or fibrosis, or a marked increase in right ventricular volume.

The pulmonary arterial pressure is normally 25/10 mm Hg. It becomes elevated when there is a large volume of pulmonary blood flow, as in a left-to-right shunt, in the presence of pulmonary vascular disease, or from an obstruction of the pulmonary venous return. Whenever it is elevated, a left atrial or wedge

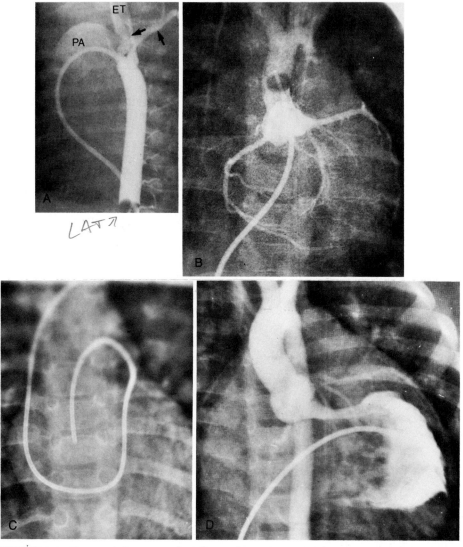

FIGURE 2–2. Characteristic course of cardiac catheter in various congenital cardiac anomalies. *A,* Patent ductus arteriosus: from the inferior vena cava through the right atrium, right ventricle, main pulmonary artery (PA), across the patent ductus arteriosus into the descending aorta. ET, Endocardial tube. *B,* Ventricular septal defect: from the inferior vena cava, through the right atrium, right ventricle, across a membranous ventricular septal defect into the ascending aorta. *C,* Aorticopulmonary window: from the inferior vena cava through the right atrium, right ventricle, main pulmonary artery, across an aorticopulmonary defect into the aortic root. *D,* Atrioventricular canal: observe the low position of the catheter across the atrial septum.

pressure must be obtained to exclude conditions such as mitral stenosis, which obstruct pulmonary venous return and cause pulmonary hypertension.

Except when stenosis occurs in the pulmonary venous system, the wedge pressure equals left atrial pressure. Left atrial pressure is elevated in mitral insufficiency, elevated left ventricular end-diastolic pressure, or mitral stenosis.

The left ventricular systolic pressure gradually increases during childhood into adulthood. An elevated left ventricular systolic pressure signifies either elevated pressure in the proximal aorta or some form of aortic stenosis. A lower than normal systolic pressure indicates shock or low cardiac output. Left ventricular diastolic pressure may be elevated because of left ventricular failure, reduced left ventricular compliance, or increased left ventricular volume.

The aortic systolic and diastolic pressures rise gradually with age. The aortic pulse pressure is generally about one third of the systolic pressure. A widened pulse pressure indicates aortic runoff, i.e., abnormal flow of blood from the aorta during diastole, as in aortic insufficiency or patent ductus arteriosus. A narrowed pulse pressure is found in patients with severe left ventricular outflow tract obstruction or low cardiac output.

When the pressure is elevated above the aortic valve, careful withdrawal pressure tracings are made around the aortic arch and through the descending aorta to exclude conditions such as supravalvular aortic stenosis or coarctation of the aorta.

Oximetric Data

Normally, oxygen saturation in the right-sided cardiac chambers is between 65 and 75 per cent with little variation between the various values, except for that of the inferior vena cava which may be greater than for other sites. A sharp increase in oxygen saturation between one chamber and the next in the right side of the heart indicates a left-to-right shunt. However, the amount of increase in oxygen saturation needed to justify a diagnosis of a left-to-right shunt becomes progressively smaller from the right atrium to the right ventricle to the pulmonary artery, since mixing improves distally. Thus, an 8 per cent increase in oxygen saturation between the venae cavae and the right atrium is necessary to diagnose a left-to-right shunt; a 5 per cent increase is necessary at the right ventricular level; and a 3 per cent increase at the arterial level.

The oxygen saturation in sites from the left side of the heart should be greater than 94 per cent. A 5 per cent decrease in oxygen saturation between the pulmonary veins and a left-sided cardiac chamber indicates a right-to-left shunt.

Derived Data

The data obtained from cardiac catheterization may be used to calculate cardiac output, volume of shunts, and vascular resistances, which are useful in assessing the severity of a condition and its effect on the circulation. The cardiac index is a valuable measurement. Normally it is 2.8 to 4.0 L/min/square meter of body surface and is the same in a newborn as in an adult.

VENTRICULAR RESPONSE TO CARDIAC ABNORMALITIES

The various cardiac conditions, whether congenital or acquired, can place increased pressure or volume loads on the cardiac chambers. The ability of the ventricles to respond to these loads influences the symptoms, signs, and radiographic findings of a patient. The response of a ventricle depends on its shape and the status of its myocardium.

At birth, both ventricles are thick-walled and round (Fig. 2–3, *left*). As the pulmonary vascular resistance and pulmonary arterial pressure fall, the right ventricle thins and becomes crescent-shaped while the left ventricle remains thick-walled and round (Fig. 2–3, *right*). The shapes and wall thickness of the ventricles influence the type of workload a ventricle can maintain. Laplace's law may be used to help understand ventricular function in response to abnormal workloads.

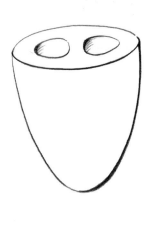
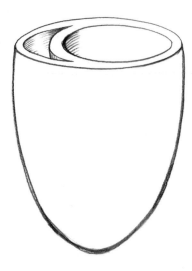

FIGURE 2–3. Diagrammatic cross-sections through the ventricles. *Left,* Newborn heart. Symmetrically appearing round muscular ventricles. *Right,* Child and adult hearts. Left ventricle round and conical, right ventricle thin-walled and crescent-shaped.

Laplace's law is T = PR, where T = tension, P = pressure, and R = radius. This law applies to a round or cylindrical object and indicates that a certain amount of tension is necessary in the wall of the object to maintain a given pressure-volume relationship. The left ventricle is round and has a relatively small radius and a large pressure (left ventricular systolic pressure). With an increase in left ventricular systolic pressure, as during a sudden episode of systemic hypertension, the change in left ventricular wall tension is relatively small, since the radius is small and the pressure is already high. This increased left ventricular systolic pressure, as in hypertension, is well maintained by the left ventricle. In contrast, when an increased volume load is placed on the left ventricle as from a left-to-right shunt or mitral insufficiency, the left ventricle dilates and its wall tension increases greatly. As the left ventricle enlarges, there is a large relative increase in the normally small radius. At this larger radius, great tension is needed to develop the normal level of left ventricular systolic pressure. In other words, the left ventricle, because of its shape, accommodates satisfactorily to elevate the left ventricular systolic pressure, but accommodates poorly to enlargement. Therefore, conditions such as aortic stenosis are well tolerated by the left ventricle, whereas abnormalities that produce large volume loads, such as patent ductus arteriosus or ventricular septal defect, are not.

The response of the right ventricle is the opposite. The right ventricle accommodates volume loads well, but does poorly with increased systolic pressure. Consider the shape and pressure of the right ventricle in older children and adults and apply Laplace's law, T = PR. Normally, the right ventricle is crescent-shaped and has a large radius (R). Right ventricular systolic pressure is low (about one fourth to one fifth of the left ventricular systolic pressure). Therefore, a volume load placed on the right ventricle, as in an atrial septal defect, is well tolerated, since the ventricle responds by increasing its already large radius. The proportional increase in radius is small; since the right ventricular systolic pressure is low, the wall tension increases only slightly. On the other hand, a sudden increase in right ventricular systolic pressure, as from the pulmonary embolus, is poorly tolerated. The normally low pressure is increased proportionally a great deal, and since the ventricle has such a large radius, it must develop a high level of wall tension to maintain the elevated pressure.

In contrast, the right ventricle of neonates is round, thick-walled, and has a small radius. It resembles a left ventricle and, therefore, can maintain high systolic pressures. In the presence of certain congenital cardiac anomalies, such as tetralogy of Fallot or transposition of the great vessels, in which the right ventricular systolic pressure is maintained at a systemic level from birth, the right ventricle retains its neonatal shape, and in essence remains hypertrophied.

The ability of a ventricle to respond to work loads also depends on the integrity of its myocardium. The development of myocardial fibrosis tends to decrease the ability of a ventricle to respond to stress. Myocardial fibrosis typically follows a myocardial infarction, but it can develop gradually in the presence of normal coronary arteries when the ventricles are chronically subjected to excessive workloads, as in aortic stenosis.

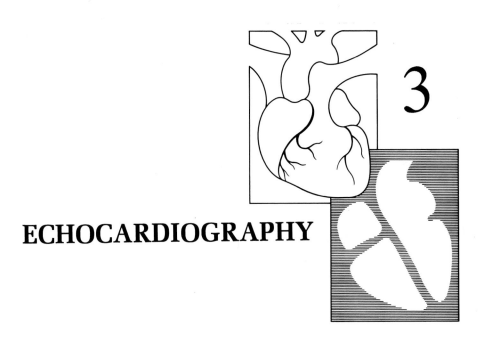

ECHOCARDIOGRAPHY

3

With the development of ultrasonic techniques, a new tool became available for the diagnosis of cardiac disease. Echocardiography has emerged as a major and important method for making cardiac diagnosis, determining disease severity, and following the course of a disease. Two forms of echocardiography are widely used, M-mode and cross-sectional.

M-MODE ECHOCARDIOGRAPHY

In M-mode echocardiography, a narrow beam of ultrasound is directed into the heart, showing the cardiac structures immediately beneath it, and a recording is made over time. Thus a single area of interest can be observed over several cardiac cycles. The direction of the echo beam can be changed, or "swept," from one area to another, in order to view additional areas, observe relations between structures, and seek continuity between structures.

Mitral Valve

The echoes from the mitral valve serve as a starting point in most echocardiographic studies. The standard transducer position along the left sternal border usually displays the anterior mitral valve leaflet well. Once it has been identified, the transducer can be rotated superiorly to identify the continuity with the posterior wall of the aorta (Fig. 3–1). Behind the anterior leaflet of the mitral valve, the movements of the posterior leaflet are seen, the former appearing as an M-shaped contour and the latter as a W-shaped contour.

FIGURE 3–1. Normal M-mode echocardiogram. Tracing through right ventricle (RV) and left ventricle (LV) showing mitral valve. Anterior leaflet of the mitral valve (AMVL) and posterior leaflet of the mitral valve (PMVL) are shown. During diastole these valves separate; during systole they come together. IVS, interventricular septum; LVPW, left ventricular posterior wall; RVAW, right ventricular anterior wall.

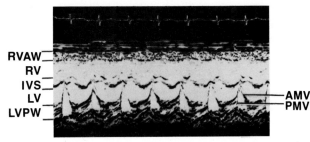

The wave forms of the anterior leaflet of the mitral valve echo can be described as:

A Point.   Peak of anterior opening motion associated with atrial contraction
B Point.   Notch on descent between the A and C points, occurring with the onset of the rise in systolic pressure
C Point.   Gradual anterior movement during ventricular systole
D Point.   Sudden onset of rapid anterior movement at the end of systole and associated with the opening of the mitral valve
E Point.   Peak of early diastolic opening movement (the most anterior position in diastole)
F Point.   Most posterior point of early diastolic closure

The movements of the posterior mitral valve are in the opposite direction and have a smaller excursion.

Particular attention is directed at two aspects of the mitral valve:

1. Leaflet excursion, increasing in mitral valve prolapse or regurgitation and decreasing in conditions such as mitral stenosis or aortic regurgitation.

2. Mitral valve diastolic closure (E-F slope), increased values found in conditions of increased flow across the mitral valve, such as ventricular septal defect, patent ductus arteriosus, and mitral insufficiency, and decreased values found in conditions of obstructed flow into the left ventricle, such as mitral stenosis or a restrictive left ventricular cardiomyopathy.

Aortic Root and Aortic Valve

As the echo beam is rotated superiorly from the mitral valve, it crosses the aortic root, which appears as two parallel dense echoes that move anteriorly during systole. The anterior echo of the aortic root is in continuity with the interventricular septum, and the posterior echo with the anterior leaflet of the mitral valve (Fig. 3–2).

The normal dimension of the aortic root ranges from 8 to 12 mm in neonates and from 20 to 40 mm in adults. The ascending aorta is dilated in conditions such as valvular aortic stenosis, aortic insufficiency, and tetralogy of Fallot.

Within the aortic root, the echoes from aortic cusps can be identified. During diastole they form a single echo in the middle of, and parallel to, the walls of the aorta. During ventricular systole, they lie along the anterior and posterior walls of the aorta.

Tricuspid Valve

Once the mitral valve has been identified, the tricuspid valve can be located by rotating the transducer medially. Usually, only the anterior leaflet is identified; since it often moves tangentially to the echo beam, it may be seen only in systole and early diastole. Its appearance is similar to that of the anterior leaflet of the mitral valve.

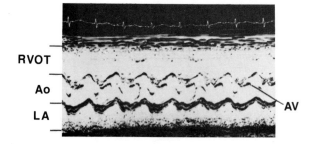

FIGURE 3–2. Normal M-mode echocardiogram. Recording through aorta (Ao), represented as parallel echoes. Within the aortic echo the aortic valve (AV) is demonstrated. Right ventricular ourflow tract (RVOT) located anteriorly and left atrium (LA) located posteriorly.

The tricuspid valvular echo is also analyzed for excursion and E-F slope. The excursion is increased in Ebstein's malformation and decreased in tricuspid stenosis. The E-F slope is increased in atrial septal defect and decreased in tricuspid stenosis or right ventricular cardiomyopathy.

Pulmonary Valve

The pulmonary valve is the structure most difficult to identify echocardiographically on an M-mode recording. Because of the angle of the pulmonary valve annulus in relation to the echo beam, only the posterior cusp is usually identified, perhaps between parallel dense echoes representing the main pulmonary artery. The appearance of the echo resembles that of an aortic valve, except that there is usually a small displacement of the valve leaflets late in diastole, immediately before the leaflets open. The small excursion, called the a-wave, corresponds with atrial contraction.

The diameter of the pulmonary root has echocardiographic values similar to those of the aortic root. The pulmonary root is enlarged in pulmonary stenosis and pulmonary hypertension and decreased in conditions with reduced pulmonary blood flow such as tetralogy of Fallot.

Left Ventricle

The left ventricle is the echo-free space in which the mitral valve is found. The interventricular septum forms its anterior margin, and the posterior left ventricular wall its posterior margin. The pericardium behind the posterior wall of the left ventricle forms rather dense echoes, particularly in comparison with those formed from the endocardium; the thickness of the posterior left ventricular wall can usually be measured easily. Measurement of the transverse diameter of the left ventricle has been used to estimate the left ventricular volume. This measurement also allows estimation of the left ventricular ejection fraction, and the velocity of shortening of the circumferential fibers (to estimate myocardial contractility). In addition, the thickness of the left ventricular posterior wall can be measured to estimate the degree of left ventricular hypertrophy.

Interventricular Septum

The interventricular septum is readily identified with the transducer placed along the left sternal border in the third and fourth intercostal spaces. It appears as a band of echoes anterior to the mitral valve, and in continuity with the anterior aortic wall (Fig. 3–3).

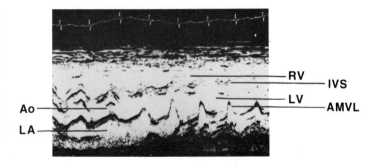

FIGURE 3–3. Normal M-mode echocardiogram. Sweep from aorta (Ao) to left ventricle (LV). Anterior leaflet of mitral valve (AMVL) continuous to posterior wall of aorta. Interventricular septum (IVS) continuous with anterior wall of aorta. Right ventricle (RV) located anteriorly to interventricular septum, and left atrium (LA) located posteriorly to aorta.

Several aspects of the interventricular septum are analyzed:

1. Septal wall motion. This is usually analyzed by observing the posterior (left ventricular) side of the interventricular septum. The various regions of the interventricular septum move differently during systole and pivot around the midpart of the septum: the superior third moves anteriorly, the middle third flattens or moves posteriorly, and the lower third moves posteriorly. Normally, the entire septum moves anteriorly at the end of systole. Abnormal (paradoxical) septal motion is found in conditions, such as atrial septal defect, which place such a volume load on the right ventricle that the septum appears to move anteriorly.

2. The thickness of the interventricular septum. It is thickened in asymmetric septal hypertrophy and other conditions that cause either left or right ventricular hypertrophy.

Right Ventricle

The right ventricle is located anteriorly to the interventricular septum. It can be difficult to distinguish the anterior wall of the right ventricle from the echoes originating from the chest wall, but often both the endocardial and epicardial surfaces can be identified (Fig. 3–3). The right ventricular dimension can be measured from the anterior wall to the interventricular septum. The right ventricular internal dimension is increased in any condition dilating the right ventricle, such as atrial septal defect. It is decreased in conditions with a hypoplastic right ventricle (tricuspid atresia), or in conditions in which the cavity is encroached upon by a hypertrophied septum, as in asymmetric septal hypertrophy.

Left Atrium

The left atrium appears as a thin-walled echo-free space behind the aortic root and mitral valve, and its posterior wall merges with the posterior left ventricular wall at the end of systole (Fig. 3–2). Observed echocardiographically, the transverse diameter of the left atrium is equal to a similar measurement of the aortic root. This ratio is increased in mitral stenosis and in conditions such as mitral insufficiency, or ventricular septal defect, where the volume of left atrial blood is increased.

Right Atrium

The right atrium and the interatrial septum cannot be assessed by M-mode echocardiography.

TWO-DIMENSIONAL ECHOCARDIOGRAPHY

In the cross-sectional form, the echo beam is quickly rotated through an arc of perhaps 70 degrees, and a wedge-shaped section of the heart and adjacent structures is recorded. These recordings are, therefore, a cross section through the heart and great vessels. The particular section obtained depends on the direction of the echo beam; there are several conventional echocardiographic projections.

Four planes are commonly used for two-dimensional echocardiographic recordings of the heart (Fig. 3–4). The first two planes are described with reference to the axis of the left ventricular outflow tract.

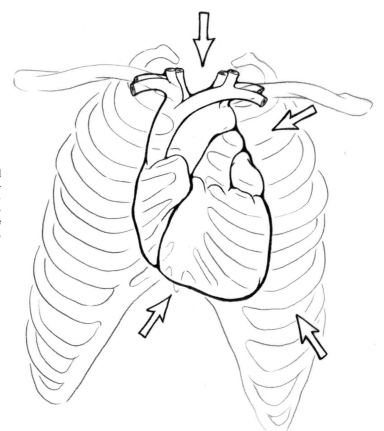

FIGURE 3–4. Four planes used for two-dimensional echocardiographic recording. Arrows indicate directions of echocardiographic planes. These are suprasternal notch, short-axis, apical, and subcostal.

1. Long-axis
2. Short-axis (perpendicular to the long-axis)
3. Oblique coronal, showing right-to-left relations and often referred to as the four-chamber view
4. Suprasternal notch

Long-Axis Plane (Fig. 3–5)

The long-axis plane may be recorded from either a left parasternal or an apical position, and a family of echocardiographic views is recorded as the transducer is angled along the chosen long-axis plane.

1. Parasternal long-axis plane. This plane, recorded along the left sternal border, shows both the inflow and outflow regions of the left ventricle, but not its apex (Fig. 3–6). In this plane, the right ventricle is located anteriorly, and both sides of the interventricular septum are imaged (Figs. 3–7 and 3–8). The sinuses of Valsalva, the aortic cusps, and the ascending aorta can be seen in this plane. Movements of both the mitral and the aortic valves can be well observed in this projection, and details of the left ventricular posterior wall and left ventricular contractility can be examined.

2. Apical long-axis plane. This is recorded with the transducer located over the apex. It allows examination of the left ventricular apex, the papillary muscle structure, and the proximal portions of the left ventricular outflow tract and the aortic valve. The latter two structures are often imaged better with this view than

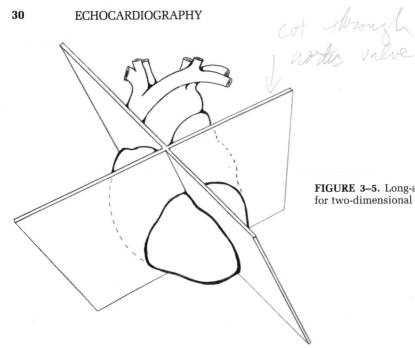

cut through
aortic valve

FIGURE 3–5. Long-axis and short-axis planes for two-dimensional echocardiography.

with parasternal projection, since they are located perpendicular to the sound waves emanating from the transducer.

These projections allow evaluation of inflow and outflow regions of the left ventricle, the configuration of the interventricular septum, the motion of the interventricular septum and posterior wall, the mitral valve anatomy, and the left atrium.

Short-Axis Plane (Fig. 3–5)

This plane is recorded in a parasternal area by rotating the transducer 90 degrees from the long-axis imaging plane. Depending on the angulation, various cross-sectional planes are recorded, not all of which are necessarily perpendicular to the left ventricular outflow tract.

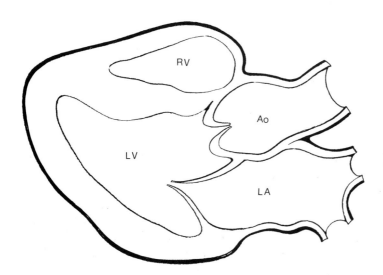

FIGURE 3–6. Parasternal long-axis plane for two-dimensional echocardiography.

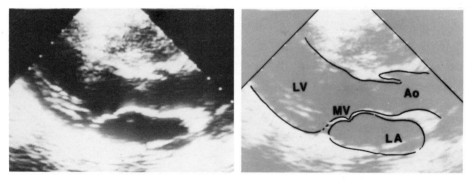

FIGURE 3–7. Two-dimensional echocardiogram. Long-axis view during systole. Mitral valve (MV) closed, aortic valve open. Ao, aorta; CT, chordae tendineae; LA, left atrium; LV, left ventricle.

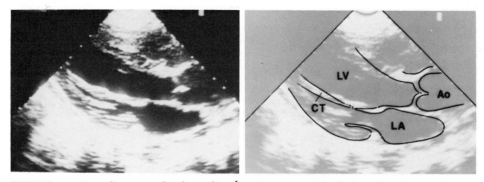

FIGURE 3–8. Two-dimensional echocardiogram. Long-axis view during diastole. Mitral valve opened, aortic valve closed. Ao, aorta; CT, chordae tendineae; LA, left atrium; LV, left ventricle.

1. Plane at the level of the great arteries (Fig. 3–9). In this projection, the aorta is seen in cross section and appears as a circle. The three aortic cusps are seen within the circle and can be observed to open and close alternately (Figs. 3–10 and 3–11). The right ventricular outflow tract and main pulmonary artery wrap around the aorta, with the pulmonary valve located at 2 o'clock. The main pulmonary artery may be seen to bifurcate into the left and the right pulmonary arteries. The right atrium is also visible, and the tricuspid valve is located at 10

FIGURE 3–9. Short-axis plane of two-dimensional echocardiogram at the level of the great arteries.

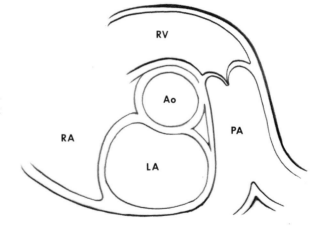

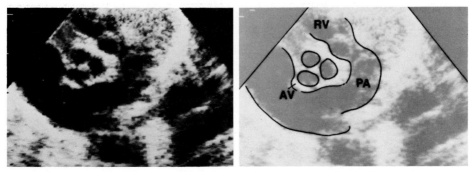

FIGURE 3–10. Two-dimensional echocardiogram. Short-axis view during diastole. Aortic valve (AV) closed. RV, right ventricle; PA, pulmonary artery.

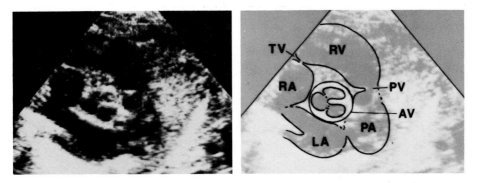

FIGURE 3–11. Two-dimensional echocardiogram. Short-axis view during systole. Tricuspid valve (TV) closed. Pulmonary valve (PV) open. LA, left atrium; PA, pulmonary artery; RA, right atrium; RV, right ventricle; AV, aortic valve.

o'clock. The atrial septum and occasionally the superior venae cavae are seen. This view is excellent for examining the aortic valve, right ventricular outflow tract, and pulmonary vein. The coronary arteries may be observed in this view.

2. Plane at the level of the mitral valve. As the transducer is swept inferiorly, the posterior leaflet of the aortic valve blends into the anterior leaflet of the mitral valve. With further inferior positioning, both leaflets of the mitral valve are imaged. During diastole, the mitral orifice appears as a "fishmouth." A cross-sectional view of both ventricles is seen, and patterns of ventricular contractility can be observed.

3. Plane at the level of the papillary muscles. A continued inferior sweep allows examination of the papillary muscles at 4 and 8 o'clock, respectively. Again, the symmetrical contractility of the left ventricle can be seen.

Apical or Subcostal Coronal Plane (Fig. 3–12)

With the transducer at the apex or in a subcostal position, a long-axis view can be obtained as discussed above. If the transducer is rotated from this plane, a family of views can be obtained. When rotated 90 degrees from the apical or subcostal position long-axis plane, an apical four-chamber view is obtained (Fig. 3–13). This view allows delineation of the inflow portions of both the right and

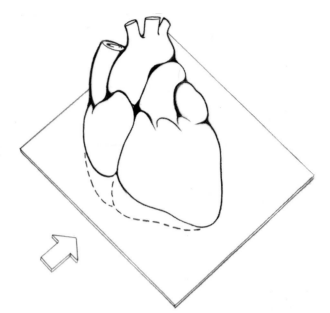

FIGURE 3–12. Plane of an oblique coronal view obtained from a subcostal projection.

left ventricles, the tricuspid and mitral valves, the ventricular and atrial septa, and, usually, the pulmonary veins entering the left atrium (Fig. 3–14). The transducer may be swept anteriorly to observe the left ventricular outflow tract and aortic valve (Fig. 3–15).

The subcostal coronal plane is recorded from a subxiphoid position and yields a coronal image similar to that of an apical projection, except that the cardiac apex is not shown.

Suprasternal Notch Plane (Fig. 3–16)

This projection, recorded with the transducer placed in the suprasternal notch, allows imaging of the great vessels and the outflow tract of the ventricles.

Because the aorta passes from anterior right to posterior left, not all of the aortic arch is visible at one time (Fig. 3–17); rather, the angulation of the transducer must be altered to show the arch in its entirety. From the aortic arch,

FIGURE 3–13. Diagram of the coronal view obtained by two-dimensional echocardiography. It is also called the four-chamber view because each of the cardiac chambers is observed.

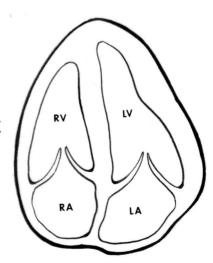

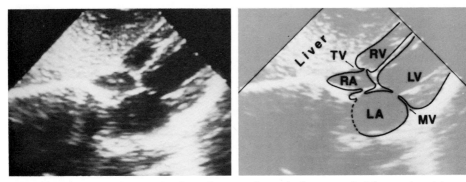

FIGURE 3–14. Two-dimensional echocardiogram. Coronal view, recorded from subcostal area. Each cardiac chamber is demonstrated. LA, left atrium; LV, left ventricle; RA, right atrium; RV, right ventricle; MV, mitral valve; TV, tricuspid valve.

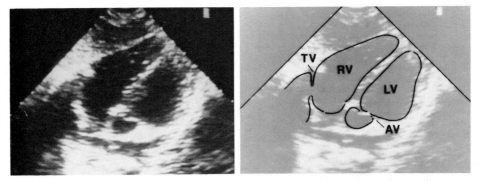

FIGURE 3–15. Two-dimensional echocardiogram. Coronal view. Subcostal recording with anterior angulation. The aortic valve (AV) and the proximal part of aorta are observed. LV, left ventricle; RV, right ventricle; TV, tricuspid valve.

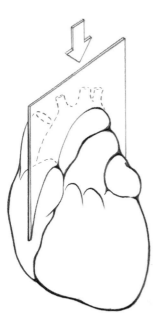

FIGURE 3–16. The suprasternal notch plane of cross-sectional echocardiography.

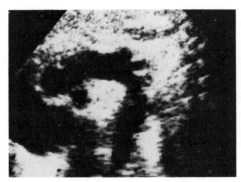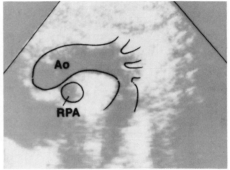

FIGURE 3–17. Two-dimensional echocardiogram. Suprasternal notch projection. Aorta (Ao) and major branches observed. Right pulmonary artery (RPA) posterior to aorta.

the innominate, left carotid, and left subclavian arteries can be seen to arise. The right pulmonary artery and the main pulmonary artery lie below the aortic arch. The left atrium may not be visible.

If the transducer is rotated 90 degrees, a suprasternal short-axis plane can be obtained. This allows a view of the superior vena cava and aortic arch. By posterior rotation, the right pulmonary artery and bifurcation from the main pulmonary artery can be seen.

Suprasternal notch views are ideal for identifying coarctation of the aorta, patent ductus arteriosus, hypoplastic ascending aorta, and transposition of the great vessels.

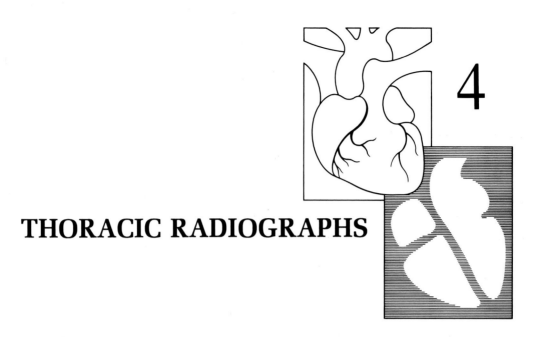

THORACIC RADIOGRAPHS

Important diagnostic information regarding the heart and major blood vessels in the thorax may be obtained through careful analysis of the thoracic radiograph. In this chapter the normal four radiographic views of the heart are discussed. Then a six-step sequence of analysis of the thorax and its content is presented, which provides an approach to cardiovascular radiographic diagnosis.

NORMAL FOUR VIEWS OF THE HEART

Four views of the heart are obtained from patients with cardiovascular disease. In each of the four views, particular cardiac structures are outlined and each view contributes in its unique way to total evaluation of the heart and its individual chambers.

Posteroanterior Projection (Figs. 4–1 and 4–2)

The right cardiac margin is formed by the right atrium and superior vena cava. The border of the right atrium extends from the diaphragm to the level of the right hilum. The superior vena cava forms a faint and straight density extending from the superior aspect of the right atrium to the level of the clavicle. In older individuals the ascending aorta forms part of the upper right cardiac border, giving it an additional convex density located along its mid-portion.

The left cardiac margin consists of four segments. The upper segment is formed by the aortic arch. This segment becomes more prominent with age. The second segment, immediately below the first, is formed by the main pulmonary artery. There is a considerable range in the appearance of a normal main pulmonary artery. The third segment is formed by the left atrial appendage, which may not be visible in a normal heart. The lowest and largest segment is formed by the left ventricle, which causes a broad convexity in this portion of the cardiac silhouette.

Lateral Projection (Figs. 4–3 and 4–4)

The lower portion of the anterior margin of the cardiac shadow is formed by the right ventricle, which is in direct contact with the sternum. Above this area of contact, the right ventricular outflow tract and the root of the main pulmonary

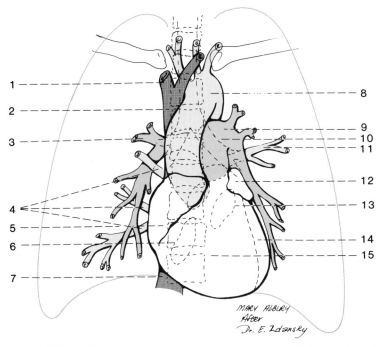

FIGURE 4–1. Diagram of the posteroanterior projection with normal pulmonary vascularity and normal cardiac size. Observe four segments of the left cardiac contour: the aortic knob, the pulmonary artery segment, the area of the left atrial appendage, and the left ventricle. The right cardiac border has three segments: the superior vena cava, the ascending aorta, and the right atrium. Note the cross sections of the bronchus and pulmonary artery in the right hilum.

1. Right innominate vein
2. Superior vena cava
3. Right main branch of the pulmonary artery
4. Upper and lower lobe veins
5. Right atrium
6. Tricuspid valve
7. Inferior vena cava
8. Arch of the aorta

9. Left main branch of the pulmonary artery
10. Main pulmonary artery
11. Left upper lobe vein
12. Appendage of the left atrium
13. Mitral valve
14. Left ventricle
15. Right ventricle

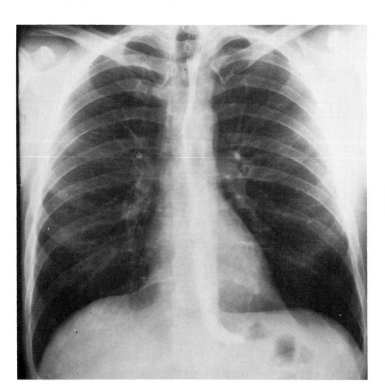

FIGURE 4–2. Normal thoracic roentgenogram in posteroanterior projection.

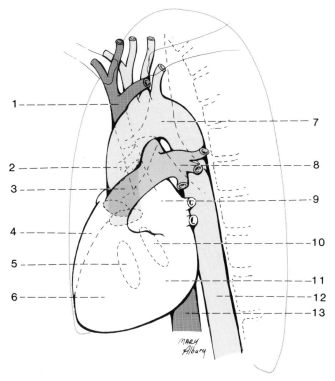

FIGURE 4–3. Diagram of the lateral projection. The retrosternal space is bound anteriorly by the sternum and posteriorly by the right ventricular outflow tract. The right ventricle and right atrium are in contact with the anterior wall of the chest. The posterior cardiac margin has three components: the left atrium, the left ventricle, and the inferior vena cava. Observe the position of the right and left pulmonary arteries.

1. Superior vena cava
2. Ascending aorta
3. Main pulmonary artery
4. Right atrium
5. Tricuspid valve
6. Right ventricle
7. Aortic arch

8. Left main branch of the pulmonary artery
9. Left atrium
10. Mitral valve
11. Left ventricle
12. Descending aorta
13. Inferior vena cava

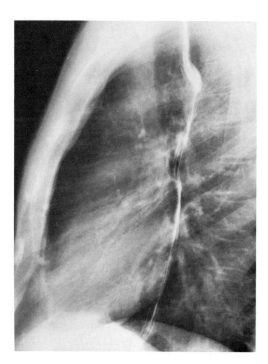

FIGURE 4–4. Normal thoracic roentgenogram in lateral projection.

artery can be seen because their anterior margin is outlined by air in the lung. The course of the pulmonary artery is superiorly and posteriorly away from the sternum. Since these structures are in contact with mediastinal fat, their margins may be indistinct, with a resulting "silhouette sign." Finally, the ascending aorta forms the uppermost segment of the anterior contour of the cardiac silhouette. The aorta courses superiorly to and blends into the superior mediastinal structures. Enlargment of either the right ventricle or ascending aorta tends to obliterate the retrosternal space (see Figs. 4–13A and 4–30).

The posterior margin of the cardiac silhouette is formed by the left atrium above and the left ventricle below. The inferior vena cava frequently forms a straight shadow immediately above the diaphragm (Fig. 4–4).

Other important anatomic landmarks can be noted on this projection. The trachea is well seen. The right pulmonary artery, as it passes directly into the right lung, is also apparent, forming a round shadow anterior to the carina.

The left pulmonary artery can also be seen; it forms a characteristic comma-shaped density as it arches over the left mainstem bronchus to enter the left lung. The left mainstem bronchus is usually seen on end.

A dark triangular space can be identified between the superior aspect of the left pulmonary artery and the inferior margin of the aortic arch.

Right Anterior Oblique Projection (Figs. 4–5 and 4–6)

In a standard 45-degree right anterior oblique projection, the posterior margin of the cardiac silhouette is formed primarily by the posterior left atrial wall. The

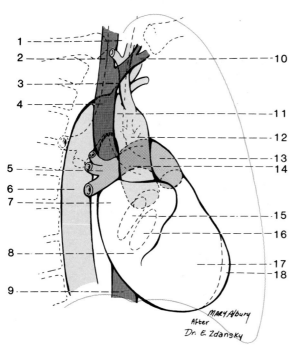

FIGURE 4–5. Diagram of the right anterior oblique projection. Segments of the anterior cardiac border are the ascending aorta, the main pulmonary artery, the right ventricular outflow tract, and the left ventricle. The posterior cardiac contour is formed by the left atrium and the right atrium.

1. Anterior wall of the trachea
2. Innominate vein
3. Anterior border of the superior vena cava
4. Superior vena cava
5. Right main branch of the pulmonary artery
6. Thoracic aorta
7. Left atrium
8. Right atrium
9. Inferior vena cava

10. Left innominate vein
11. Arch of the aorta
12. Left main branch of the pulmonary artery
13. Main stem of the pulmonary artery
14. Left main bronchus
15. Tricuspid valve
16. Mitral valve
17. Right ventricle
18. Left ventricle

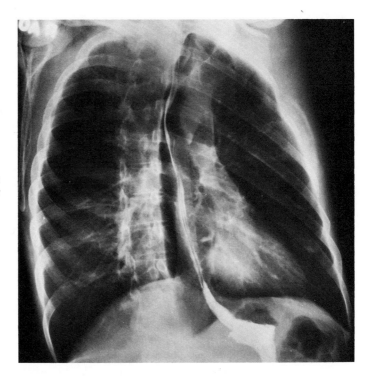

FIGURE 4–6. Normal thoracic roentgenogram in right anterior oblique projection.

right atrium forms the lowermost part of the posterior margin. The inferior vena cava or the hepatic veins, or both, frequently cast a straight shadow immediately above the diaphragm.

Anteriorly, the uppermost convexity represents the anterior wall of the ascending aorta, below which the main pulmonary artery and the right ventricular outflow tract are evident. The lower segment is markedly convex and formed almost exclusively by the right ventricle. Occasionally, part of the apex of the left ventricle may partially contribute to the formation of this segment. With lesser degrees of obliquity, the right atrium and left ventricle form a larger part of the lower segments of the posterior and anterior margins, respectively. In this projection the aortic arch and the left pulmonary artery are seen on end.

Left Anterior Oblique Projection (Figs. 4–7 and 4–8)

Depending on the degree of obliquity, the anterior cardiac border is formed by either the right ventricle or the right atrium. The posterior margin is convex and formed by the left atrium above and left ventricle below. In the 55- to 60-degree projection, this margin does not normally overlie the spine posteriorly.

Other important structures well demonstrated in this projection are the ascending aorta, which forms the upper margin of the anterior segment, and the space between the aortic arch and pulmonary artery. The trachea and left mainstem bronchus are well seen. The relationship of the left pulmonary artery above, and left atrium below the left mainstem bronchus, can be seen with proper radiographic technique.

PLAIN FILM DIAGNOSIS OF CARDIAC DISEASE

One way to approach the radiographic diagnosis of cardiac disease is to analyze each case in a series of six steps.

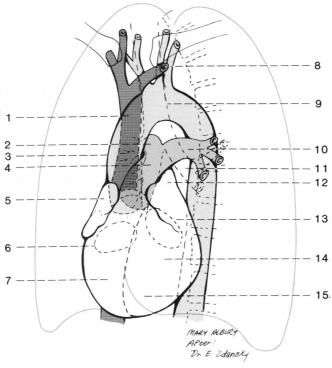

FIGURE 4–7. Diagram of the left anterior oblique projection. The anterior cardiac contour has the following segments: the ascending aorta, the right atrium, and the right atrial appendage. The posterior cardiac contour is formed by the left atrium and the left ventricle.

1. Superior vena cava
2. Right main branch of the pulmonary artery
3. Ascending aorta
4. Main pulmonary artery
5. Right atrial appendage
6. Tricuspid valve
7. Right ventricle
8. Left subclavian artery

9. Posterior border of the trachea
10. Left main branch of the pulmonary artery
11. Left main bronchus
12. Left atrium
13. Mitral valve
14. Left ventricle
15. Inferior vena cava

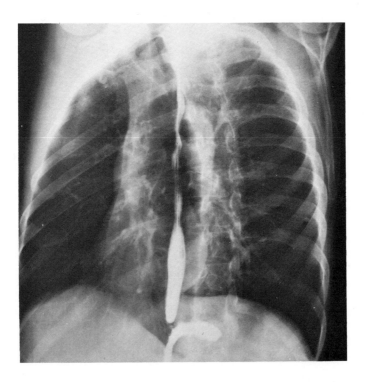

FIGURE 4–8. Thoracic roentgenogram in left anterior oblique projection.

1. *Evaluation of the Thoracic Cage for Signs of Previous Surgery or Other Abnormalities*

Most corrective cardiac operations are performed through a midline sternotomy. Postoperative wire sutures about the sternum are generally seen, and on a lateral view there is evidence of periosteal elevation. Patent ductus arteriosus, coarctation repair, and left-sided Blalock-Taussig procedures are performed through a left thoracotomy; the right-sided Blalock-Taussig, the Waterston shunt, the Glenn procedure, and the Blalock-Hanlon atrial septostomy are performed through a right thoracotomy. Occasionally, a rib is resected for this thoracotomy, but this operative approach is usually recognized by asymmetry of the thoracic cage with a smaller, and slightly deformed, rib at the site of the thoracotomy.

The incidence of bony abnormalities of the thorax in patients with congenital heart disease is high. Premature fusion of the sternum is commonly observed in patients with cyanotic forms of congenital cardiac anomalies (Fig. 4–9). Hypersegmentation of the sternum occurs with increased frequency in Down's syndrome (Fig. 4–10). A markedly enlarged right ventricle, as occurs in atrial septal defect, causes bulging of the sternum (Fig. 4–11).

The lower margins of ribs are notched in conditions with enlarged intercostal arteries serving as collateral vessels (Fig. 4–12). Although typical in older patients with coarctation of the aorta, they also develop following Blalock-Taussig shunts, being unilateral in these cases.

Spinal abnormalities such as hemivertebrae or scoliosis are frequently observed in patients with congenital cardiac anomalies. Postoperative sternal and rib changes can be seen following correction or palliative procedures.

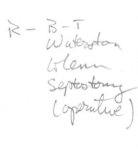

2. *Identification of the Position of the Stomach Bubble and Hepatic Shadow to Determine Body Sites*

The stomach bubble should be located in the left upper quadrant and the hepatic shadow in the right upper quadrant. In patients with congenital cardiac

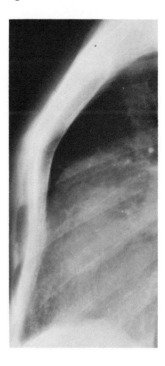

FIGURE 4–9. Complete fusion of sternal segments.

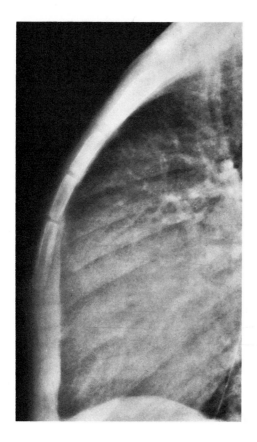

FIGURE 4–10. Hypersegmentation of the sternum in a patient with Down's syndrome.

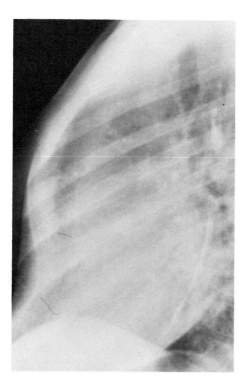

Allow 1/3 space for ne retrosternally

FIGURE 4–11. Atrial septal defect with enlarged right ventricle and anterior bulging of the sternum.

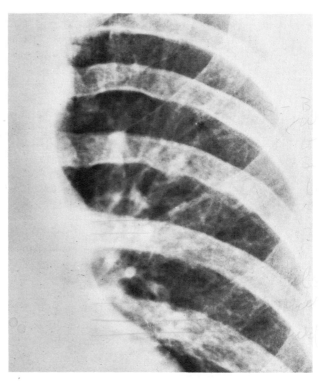

FIGURE 4–12. Notching of the inferior rib margin in coarctation of the aorta.

atria ↔ situs
AV valves ↔ ventricles

anomalies, abnormalities in position of the viscera, which are often recognized by abnormal hepatic and stomach position, may be present. The diagnostic approach to such problems is discussed in the chapters on congenital heart disease.

3. Evaluation of Great Vessels for Size and Position

Enlargement of the Pulmonary Artery Segment. When the pulmonary artery is in a normal position, its enlargement results in a prominent pulmonary arterial segment along the left upper cardiac border. The pulmonary artery is in an abnormal position in transposition of great vessels and some cases of truncus arteriosus; the pulmonary arterial segment of the posteroanterior cardiac contour is concave even in the presence of markedly increased pulmonary blood flow.

Enlargement of the Aorta. Three portions of the aorta can be evaluated radiographically: ascending aorta, aortic arch, and descending aorta. Usually, the ascending aorta does not extend beyond the right upper mediastinal shadow. Enlargement of the ascending aorta tends to obliterate the retrosternal space (Fig. 4–13). In patients with a left aortic arch, the aortic arch passes obliquely, anteriorly to posteriorly, to the left of the trachea and esophagus and displaces them slightly to the right (Fig. 4–14). In patients with an enlarged aortic arch, the aortic knob is more prominent and the trachea displaced more to the right. The position of the aortic arch can be established by observing the relationship of the supracardiac portion of the barium-filled esophagus with the trachea, since the esophagus maintains a constant relationship with the aortic arch and descending aorta. Therefore, if the barium column is seen to the left of the trachea, it is a left arch, and vice versa (Fig. 4–15). The descending aorta forms a slightly convex density alongside the spine. In the elderly with ectasia of the aorta, the descending aorta is more prominent and displaces the barium-filled esophagus posteriorly to the left.

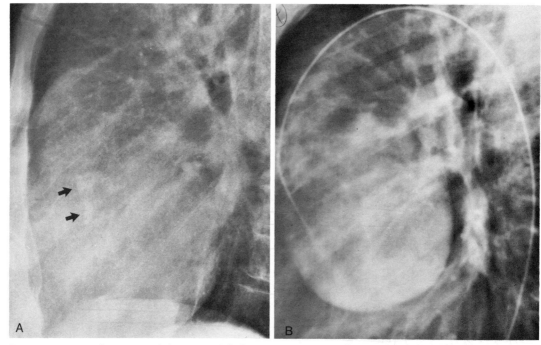

FIGURE 4–13. Enlargement of the aorta. Calcific aortic stenosis and secondary cystic medial necrosis. *A*, Thoracic roentgenogram, lateral projection. Obliteration of the retrosternal space by markedly dilated ascending aorta. Calcifications in the area of the aortic valve (arrows). *B*, Aortogram in a patient with Marfan's disease. Massive dilatation of the aortic sinuses and ascending aorta.

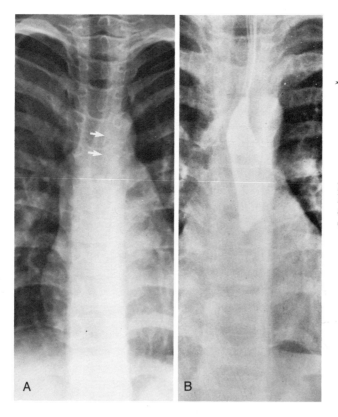

FIGURE 4–14. Left aortic arch. *A*, Aortic knob indents and displaces the tracheal air column (arrows) to the right. *B*, Barium column to the left of the trachea.

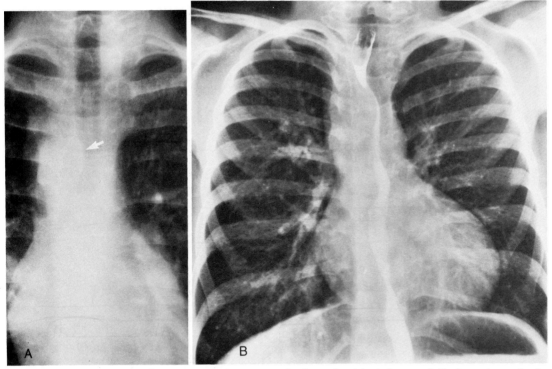

FIGURE 4–15. Right aortic arch. *A*, Aortic knob on the right indents and displaces the tracheal air column to the left (arrow). *B*, Barium column overlies and is slightly to the right of the trachea and follows the aortic arch and descending aorta.

4. Evaluation of Specific Chamber Enlargement

Enlargement of each cardiac chamber can be evaluated radiographically using the various projections. The size of the left atrium can be assessed with the most reliability.

Signs of Left Atrial Enlargement. Several features allow recognition of left atrial enlargement on a posteroanterior projection:

1. The barium-filled esophagus below the carina is commonly displaced toward the right (Fig. 4–16*A*), since left atrial dilatation occurs posteriorly and superiorly to the right (Figs. 4–16*B* and *C*), although, when it is massively dilated, it also extends into the left side (Fig. 4–16*D*) and can, therefore, displace the barium column to the left.

2. The left atrial appendage forms a prominent bulge along the mid-left cardiac border (Fig. 4–17).

3. A double density is noted along the right cardiac border (Fig. 4–17). A similar appearance may be found in patients with a normal-sized left atrium or a confluence of pulmonary veins (Fig. 4–18).

4. Widening of the angle of the carina is caused by the elevation of the left mainstem bronchus by the enlarged left atrium (Fig. 4–19).

In the lateral projection, a left atrial enlargement is recognized by posterior displacement of both walls of the barium-filled esophagus (Fig. 4–20). Normally, the anterior wall of the esophagus may be indented, but not both walls (Fig. 4–21). Occasionally, there is no indentation of the esophagus by a very large left atrium. This phenomenon has been called esophageal escape (Fig. 4–22).

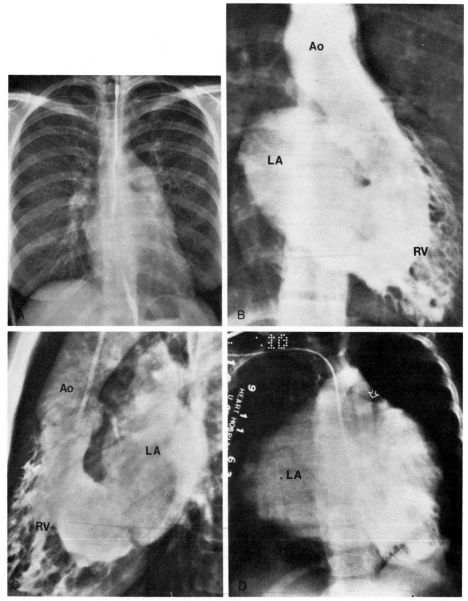

FIGURE 4–16. A, Left atrial enlargement evident by a double density in the area of the left atrium, prominent left atrial appendage, and slight displacement of the barium column to the right. Normal pulmonary vascularity and cardiac size. B, Angiogram. Anteroposterior projection. Injection in inverted right ventricle (RV). Aorta opacifies (Ao). Massive mitral regurgitation. LA, Left atrium. C, Angiogram. Lateral projection. Injection in an anatomic right ventricle. Massive mitral regurgitation. D, Left ventriculogram. Posteroanterior projection. Massive mitral regurgitation. Dilated left atrium (LA). Elevation and compression of the left mainstem bronchus (open arrow).

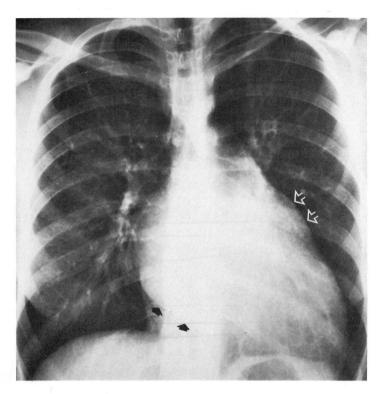

FIGURE 4–17. Left atrial enlargement evidenced by double density (arrows) and prominent left atrial appendage (white arrows). Prominent vascular markings in the upper lobes. Cardiomegaly. Left ventricular enlargement with downward displacement of the apex. Prominent main pulmonary artery segment.

In the left anterior oblique projection, an enlarged left atrium elevates the left mainstem bronchus and obliterates the spaces between the posterior cardiac margin and the left mainstem bronchus (Fig. 4–23).

Signs of Left Ventricular Enlargement. In the posterior anterior projection, several features of left ventricular enlargement can be observed.

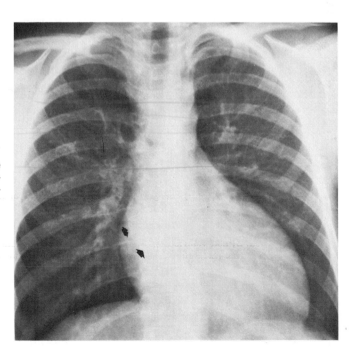

FIGURE 4–18. Double density in the area of the left atrium (arrows) corresponding to a pulmonary venous confluence.

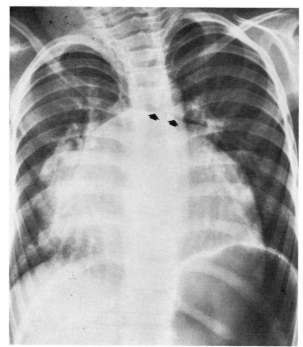

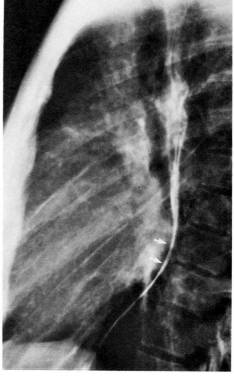

FIGURE 4–19. A massively dilated left atrium elevates and narrows the left mainstem bronchus (arrows). Cardiomegaly.

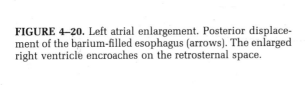

FIGURE 4–20. Left atrial enlargement. Posterior displacement of the barium-filled esophagus (arrows). The enlarged right ventricle encroaches on the retrosternal space.

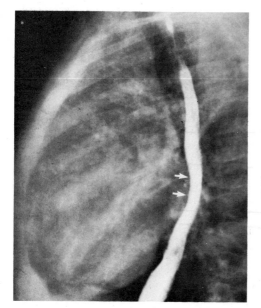

FIGURE 4–21. The anterior wall of the esophagus (arrows) is displaced by an enlarged left atrium during diastole.

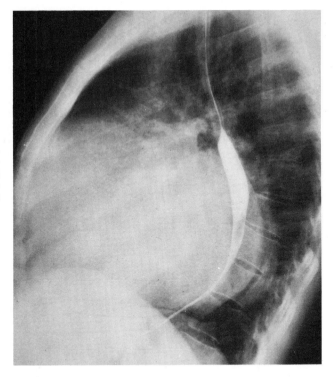

FIGURE 4–22. The enlarged left atrium has gone beyond the barium-filled esophagus, which is posteriorly displaced (esophageal escape). Marked cardiomegaly. Obliteration of the retrosternal space by the enlarged right ventricle.

1. Left ventricular dilatation produces downward displacement of the apex toward the diaphragm (Fig. 4–24A).

2. Left ventricular hypertrophy produces a round left cardiac border (Fig. 4–25A).

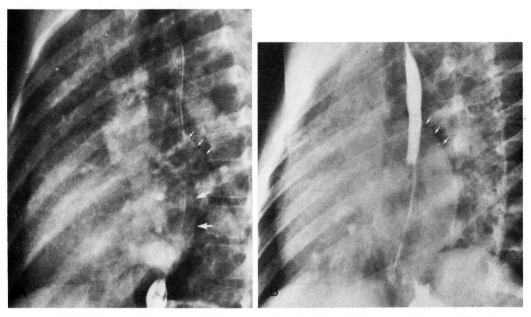

FIGURE 4–23. Left anterior oblique projections. A, Normal. Dark space between left mainstem bronchus (small white arrows) and cardiac contour (large white arrows). B, Severe mitral insufficiency. Left atrial enlargement. Obliteration of space by a dilated left atrium. Left bronchus (white arrows).

LAO good for LA, LV

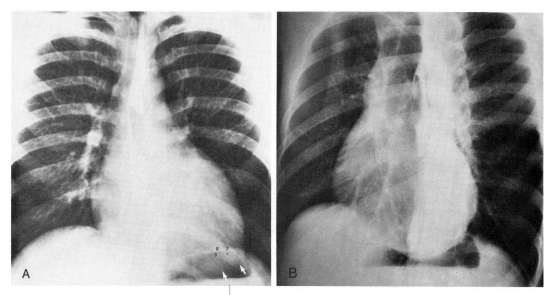

FIGURE 4–24. Left ventricular enlargement. A, Posteroanterior projection. Downward displacement of the cardiac apex, seen through gastric gas bubble (arrows). Normal pulmonary vascularity. Cardiomegaly. B, Left anterior oblique projection. Posterior and downward displacement of the cardiac apex indenting the gastric fundus. The cardiac shadow markedly overlaps the spine.

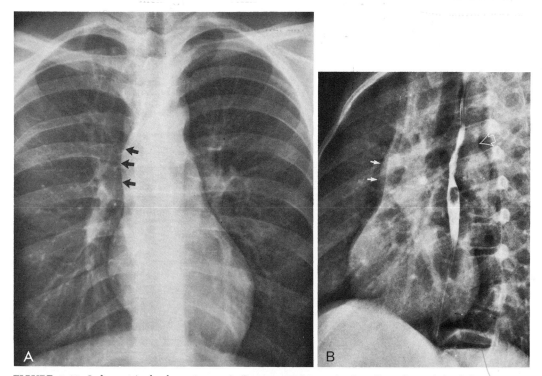

FIGURE 4–25. Left ventricular hypertropy. A, Posteroanterior projection. Rounding of the left cardiac border. Normal pulmonary vascularity and cardiac size. Prominence of the ascending aorta (arrows). B, Left anterior oblique projection. The enlarged left ventricle overlaps the anterior margin of vertebral bodies. Prominent ascending aorta (arrows). Coarctation of the aorta and poststenotic dilatation (open arrow).

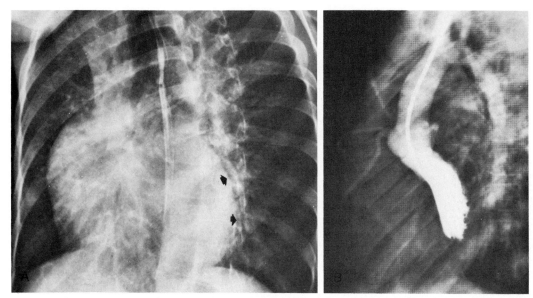

FIGURE 4–26. Right ventricular enlargement mimicking left ventricular enlargement. *A*, Left anterior oblique projection. Prominent right cardiac border indicates either right ventricular or atrial enlargement. Left ventricular border (arrows) displaced by the enlarged right side of the heart. *B*, Left ventriculogram. Lateral projection. Posterior displacement and elevation of the left ventricle by the enlarged right ventricle.

In a left anterior oblique projection, left ventricular enlargement causes the posterior cardiac margin to overlap the vertebral column (Figs. 4–24*B* and 4–25*B*). Right ventricular enlargement displacing the left ventricle posteriorly (Fig. 4–26), or a shallow left anterior obliquity (Fig. 4–27) in a normal patient, can mimic left ventricular enlargement.

Signs of Right Atrial Enlargement. It is difficult to accurately predict right atrial enlargement radiographically. It does cause an increased convexity of the lower right heart border on the posteroanterior projection (Fig. 4–28).

Signs of Right Ventricular Enlargement. In patients suspected of having

FIGURE 4–27. Shallow left anterior oblique projection. The posterior cardiac contour overlaps the spine (arrow), simulating left ventricular enlargement.

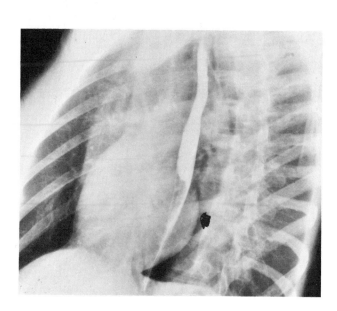

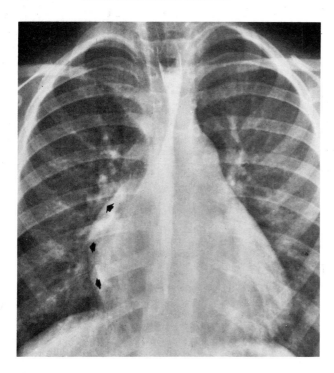

FIGURE 4–28. Complete endocardial cushion defect. Right atrial enlargement evidenced by increased convexity of the lower right cardiac border (arrows). Increased pulmonary vascularity and cardiomegaly.

cardiac disease, rounding and elevation of the cardiac apex suggest right ventricular enlargement (Fig. 4–29). In the lateral projection, the retrosternal space is obliterated by right ventricular dilatation (Fig. 4–30). In the left anterior oblique projection, increased convexity of the anterior cardiac border is indicative of right heart enlargement (Fig. 4–26A).

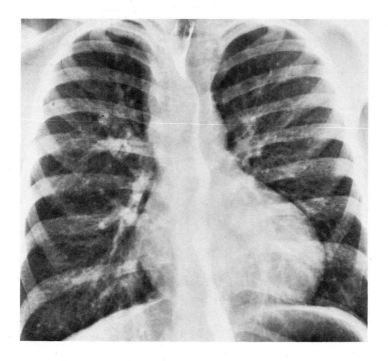

FIGURE 4–29. Round, elevated cardiac apex. Right aortic arch. Bizarre pulmonary vascular pattern with multiple vascular cross sections and unusual distribution of vascular markings. Heart slightly enlarged.

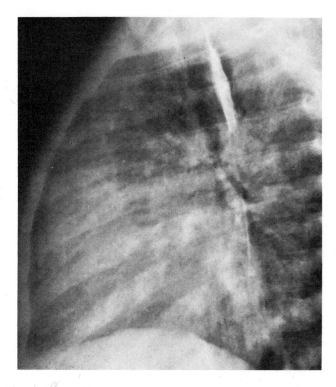

FIGURE 4–30. Obliteration of the retrosternal space by an enlarged right ventricle. Enlarged pulmonary arteries. Cardiomegaly.

55–60% in
1ˢᵗ yr of life

5. Evaluation of Cardiac Size and Contour

Cardiomegaly indicates an increase in the volume of blood within the heart, and rarely an increase in muscle mass (hypertrophy). The neonatal cardiac silhouette normally appears larger in comparison to the thoracic cage than that of an adult. One index of cardiac enlargement is the cardiothoracic ratio, which in infants may be 0.55 in contrast to normal upper limit of 0.45 in adults. In evaluation of cardiac size, the lateral and oblique views must be considered when assessing the diameter of the heart in an anteroposterior direction (see Figs. 4–2, 4–4, 4–6, and 4–8).

There are certain cardiac contours that are very diagnostic of chamber enlargement, as just discussed, or of a specific cardiac condition. The latter will be discussed in the appropriate sections.

6. Evaluation of Pulmonary Vascularity

Pulmonary vascularity can give clues about the volume of pulmonary blood flow, can reflect the level of pulmonary venous pressure, and, at times, can reveal abnormal sources of pulmonary blood flow. The analysis of pulmonary vascularity provides important information for the evaluation of cardiac disease, whether congenital or acquired.

In a normal thoracic radiograph, the pulmonary vascular markings taper gradually toward the peripheral of the lung fields (Fig. 4–31). Most of the vascular densities that are seen are caused primarily by pulmonary arteries and not by pulmonary veins. The vascular markings are more prominent in the lower lung fields. The vessels in the right hilum appear to be larger than those in the left, because the left hilum is partially overshadowed by the cardiac silhouette.

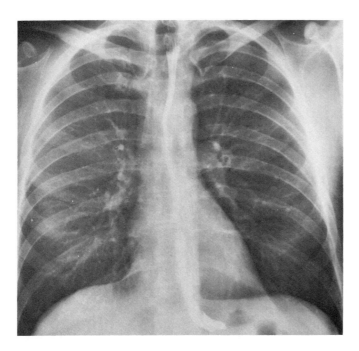

FIGURE 4–31. Gradual tapering of pulmonary vascular markings from the hilum toward the periphery of the lung. Cross sections through a bronchus and a vessel are seen in the hilum.

Six different vascular patterns are recognized.

1. Normal pulmonary vascularity (Fig. 4–31). The right and left main pulmonary arteries are of normal caliber and taper gradually through the middle third of the lung fields. Scant pulmonary vascular markings are present in the outer third. Normal pulmonary vascularity is present in (a) a normal heart, (b) obstructive lesions of either the right or left side of the heart, and (c) conditions with either a small left-to-right or a small right-to-left shunt.

2. Increased pulmonary vascularity due to increased pulmonary blood flow in

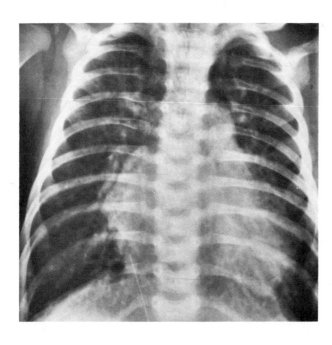

FIGURE 4–32. Left-to-right shunt. Indistinct vascular markings. Cardiomegaly. Prominent main pulmonary artery segment. Left aortic arch.

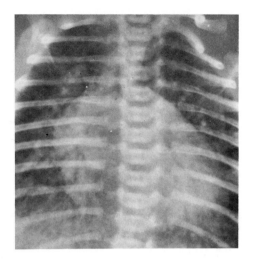

FIGURE 4–33. Cardiomegaly. Concave pulmonary artery segment. Markedly increased pulmonary vascularity.

conditions with left-to-right shunts (Fig. 4–32), or admixture lesions (Fig. 4–33). The main pulmonary artery and hilar arteries are prominent, and the peripheral arteries are sharply outlined and dilated and are distributed equally to both the upper and lower lobes. The pulmonary vascular markings do not accurately reflect the volume of pulmonary blood flow. Increased pulmonary arterial vasculature is present in (a) conditions, such as ventricular septal defect or patent ductus arteriosus, associated with a left-to-right shunt (Fig. 4–32) and (b) admixture lesions, such as truncus arteriosus (Fig. 4–33) or transposition of the great vessels, with both a left-to-right and right-to-left shunt.

3. Decreased pulmonary vascularity due to right-to-left shunts. The main pulmonary arterial segment may be small, but more commonly the diameter of the hilar pulmonary arteries is reduced, and these taper rapidly so that the lung fields appear dark (Fig. 4–34). Decreased pulmonary arterial vascular markings occur in conditions such as tetralogy of Fallot or tricuspid atresia, with an intracardiac defect, and obstruction to pulmonary blood flow (usually pulmonary stenosis).

4. Pulmonary venous congestion. A pattern of increased pulmonary venous vascularity, or pulmonary venous obstruction, occurs in any condition that causes increased resistance distal to pulmonary capillaries (Fig. 4–35). Mitral stenosis and acute left ventricular failure are two common causes.

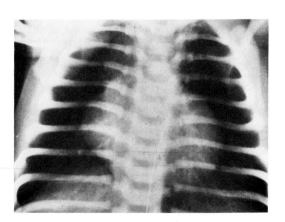

FIGURE 4–34. Tricuspid atresia. Decreased pulmonary vascularity. Cardiomegaly. Round upturned cardiac apex.

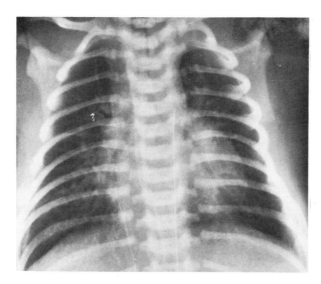

FIGURE 4–35. Hypoplastic left heart. Increased pulmonary vascularity with a congestive pattern. Cardiomegaly. Prominent right cardiac border.

In the early stage of pulmonary venous hypertension, there is constriction of the lower lobe pulmonary veins radiographically. When the pulmonary venous pressure exceeds 25 mm Hg (the plasma osmotic pressure), fluid accumulates in the interstitial tissues and Kerley B lines appear. At this point, the hilar vessels become prominent and indistinct, and a cuff of edema may appear around the bronchi in the hilar region (Fig. 4–36). As the venous pressure increases to more than 30 to 35 mm Hg, there is frank alveolar edema and pleural effusion. Elevated pulmonary venous pressure can be identified roentgenologically in only about 60 per cent of cases. This lack of correlation between the level of the pulmonary venous pressure and the appearance of the pulmonary vasculature is one of the limitations of the roentgenologic diagnosis of cardiac disease.

5. Bronchial collaterals (Fig. 4–37). Discrete pulmonary arteries are not found in the hila, and there are vascular shadows entering the medial portions of the lungs at other locations. Frequently these follow a tortuous course.

6. A bizarre pattern of pulmonary vascularity, usually with a different vascular pattern in each lung. This is evident radiographically when (a) the pattern of pulmonary vascularity is different between the two lungs (Fig. 4–38), or (b) there is an abnormal pulmonary vascular shadow in one lung (Fig. 4–39). Pulmonary vascularity should also be evaluated for a pattern of pulmonary edema.

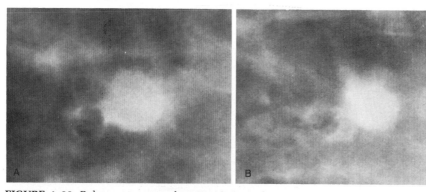

FIGURE 4–36. Pulmonary venous hypertension. *A,* Cross section of bronchus and pulmonary vessel in the right hilum in absence of interstitial fluid. *B,* Cross section of bronchus and pulmonary vessels showing extensive peribronchial cuffing. Indistinct markings of both bronchus and vessel.

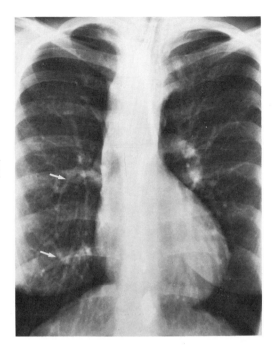

FIGURE 4–37. Abnormal distribution of pulmonary vessels, particularly in the right lung (arrows). Round upturned cardiac apex. Right aortic arch.

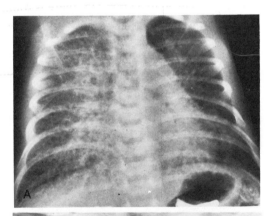

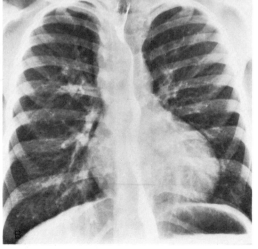

FIGURE 4–38. Asymmetrical pulmonary vascular markings. *A,* Stenosis of right pulmonary veins. Increased pulmonary vascular markings. Reticular pattern in the right lung. *B,* Pulmonary atresia. Asymmetry of vascular markings. Large bronchial collateral arteries to the right lung.

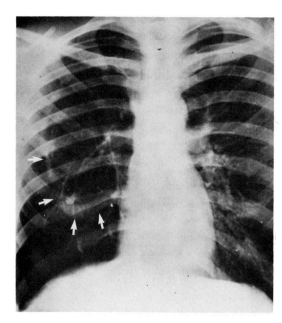

FIGURE 4–39. Anomalous course of a normally connected pulmonary vein (arrows).

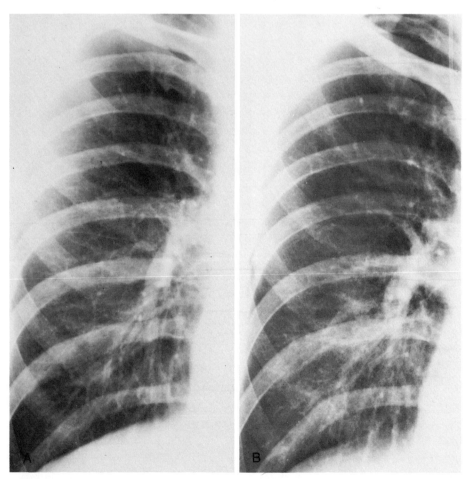

FIGURE 4–40. *A*, Normal. Distinctly seen vascular markings in the lower lobe. *B*, Indistinctness of vascular markings in lower lobe caused by increased interstitial fluid.

Pulmonary Vascularity in Left-Sided Failure

Six factors influence the distribution of pulmonary blood flow. Three of these factors remain constant throughout the lungs. Interstitial osmotic and alveolar pressures are constant. The osmotic pressure is about 25 to 30 mm Hg; alveolar pressure plays a role in regulating capillary blood flow. An elevation of alveolar pressure, as in asthma, causes a diminution of the caliber of alveolar capillaries and an increase in pulmonary vascular resistance.

The other three factors—hydrostratic, pulmonary arterial, and pulmonary venous pressures—diminish from base to apex because of gravitational effects. The normal distribution of pulmonary blood flow produces relative underperfusion of the upper lobes and overperfusion of the lower lobes.

In the presence of left-sided cardiac failure from any cause, the increased pulmonary venous pressure resulting from the elevated left ventricular end-diastolic pressure causes an imbalance among the factors regulating pulmonary blood flow. The transudation of fluid into the pulmonary interstitium causes an increase in the interstitial pressure, which leads to a constriction of the lower lobe pulmonary arterioles, increasing the pulmonary vascular resistance in this region. Blood is then redistributed to the upper lobes.

The earliest radiographic manifestation of left-sided cardiac failure is an indistinctness of the vascular markings caused by the presence of increased interstitial fluids, especially at the lung bases (Fig. 4–40). The hilar vessels become

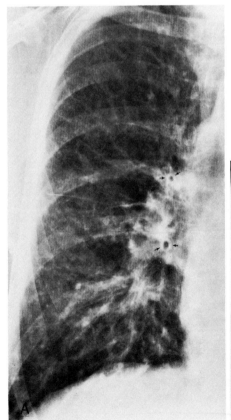
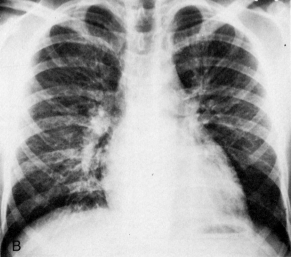

FIGURE 4–41. Left-sided cardiac failure. *A,* Indistinct vascular markings in lower lobe. Kerley B lines. Peribronchial cuffing from interstitial fluid (arrows). *B,* Indistinctness of vascular markings in lower lobes. Redistribution of blood flow toward upper lobes. Cardiomegaly.

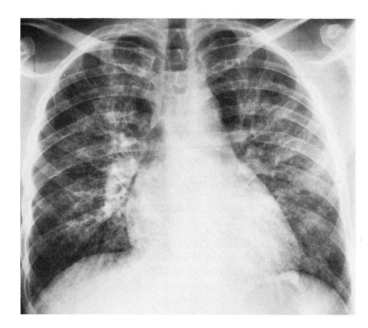

FIGURE 4–42. Small bilateral pleural effusions. Diffuse interstitial and alveolar infiltrates in both lung fields, predominantly in the upper lobes. Cardiac size at upper limits of normal.

enlarged and indistinct. The increased interstitial fluid can also be seen as "peribronchial" cuffing (Fig. 4–36 and 4–41A). Later, "cephalization" occurs. This indicates that the vascular markings are prominent in the upper lobes owing to the constriction of the lower lobe vessels and redistribution of flow to the upper lobes (Fig. 4–41B).

Pleural effusion occurs late and is more prominent on the right side than on the left. Cardiac size is almost invariably increased in cardiac failure (Fig. 4–42).

Transudation of fluid into the alveoli leads to pulmonary edema. This appears in a perihilar location, yielding the radiographic appearance called "butterfly wings" or "bat wings" (Fig. 4–43A), but the peripheral lung fields are clear except in severe cases when the entire lung fields are consolidated (Fig. 4–43B). Kerley

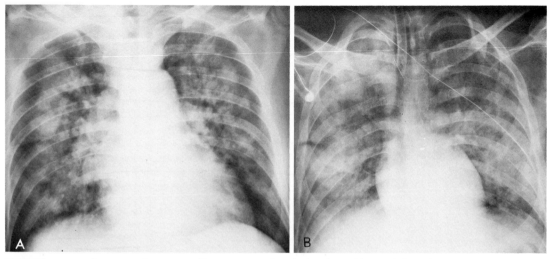

FIGURE 4–43. Pulmonary edema. A, Diffuse interstitial and alveolar infiltrates bilaterally with "butterfly wings" appearance. B, Extensve consolidation of both lungs.

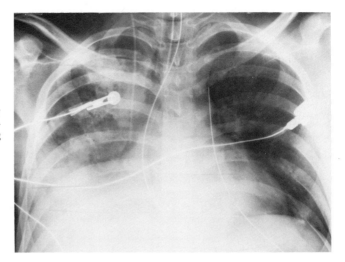

FIGURE 4–44. Unilateral pulmonary edema. Extensive interstitial and alveolar infiltrates in right lung. Left lung clear.

B lines, due to fluid in the interlobular septum, are also seen in long-standing pulmonary edema.

Pulmonary edema usually involves both lungs, but unilateral or focal pulmonary edema occurs if the interstitial or hydrostatic pressure is different between the lungs, as in patients with orthostatic unilateral pulmonary edema (Fig. 4–44) or with obstructive pulmonary disease, in which pulmonary edema occurs in areas with functioning pulmonary tissue (Fig. 4–45).

Several noncardiac causes, with various physiologic mechanisms, must be considered in the differential diagnosis of pulmonary edema:

1. Uremia. Increased capillary permeability.
2. Fluid overload. Decreased plasma osmotic pressure.
3. Neurogenic. Altered capillary permeability or capillary pressure.
4. Hypoproteinemia. Decreased plasma osmotic pressure.
5. Transfusion and allergic reactions. Altered capillary permeability.
6. Inhalation of toxic gases. Altered capillary permeability.

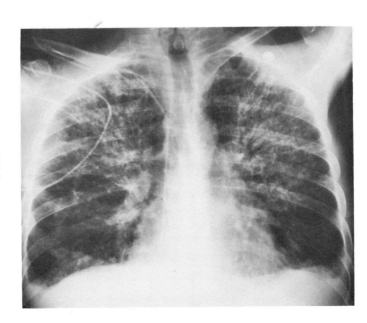

FIGURE 4–45. Focal areas of pulmonary edema involving predominantly the upper lobes in a patient with chronic obstructive pulmonary disease.

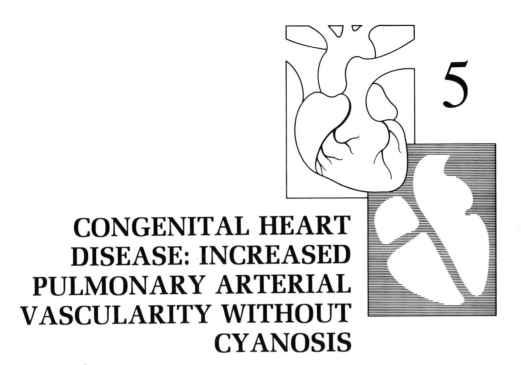

CONGENITAL HEART DISEASE: INCREASED PULMONARY ARTERIAL VASCULARITY WITHOUT CYANOSIS

Congenital heart disease may be classified in various ways. In this book we will discuss the roentgenographic diagnosis of congenital heart disease using a physiologic approach described by Lester and coworkers. It is based on the radiographic appearance of the pulmonary vasculature and the presence or absence of cyanosis. This approach may also be extended to the diagnosis of acquired heart disease. With some experience, the radiologist is able to decide whether the vasculature is normal, decreased, increased, or bizarre, thus categorizing the lesion physiologically. From this point, he can further analyze cardiac size, chamber enlargement, and position and size of the great vessels for more precise diagnosis.

Increased pulmonary arterial vascularity in an acyanotic patient indicates the presence of a left-to-right shunt and increased pulmonary blood flow. The pulmonary vascularity is not necessarily proportional to the volume of shunt, paticularly in patients with increased pulmonary blood flow associated with a decreased pulmonary vascular resistance. For instance, a patient with an atrial septal defect may have a 60 per cent shunt with normal cardiac contour and pulmonary vascularity, while a comparable shunt in a patient with a ventricular septal defect will have increased pulmonary vascularity, since the latter is usually associated with pulmonary hypertension. Similarly, a small-sized shunt (20 to 30 per cent) at the ventricular or great vessel level is associated with normal pulmonary vascularity. Therefore, a left-to-right shunt at the atrial level, or small shunt at the ventricular level, cannot be diagnosed on the basis of normal chest films.

The next diagnostic step is to evaluate left atrial size. Congenital cardiac anomalies classified as left-to-right shunt lesions may be divided into two groups, according to the presence or absence of left atrial enlargement, indicating that the left-to-right shunt occurs proximally or distally to the mitral valve, respectively.

65

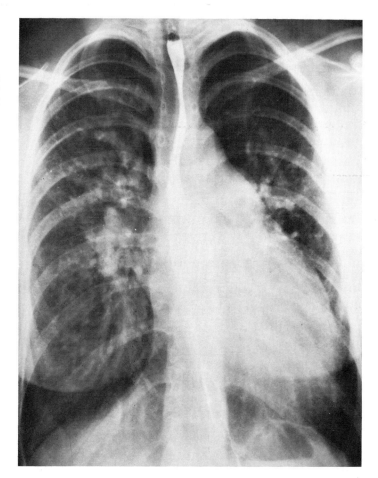

PDA

FIGURE 5–1. Extracardiac shunt due to patent ductus arteriosus. Increased pulmonary arterial vascularity. Cardiomegaly with downward displacement of the apex. Large aortic knob. Prominent pulmonary artery segment.

VSD

FIGURE 5–2. Intracardiac shunt due to ventricular septal defect. Increased pulmonary arterial vascularity. Cardiomegaly. Small aortic arch. Large pulmonary artery.

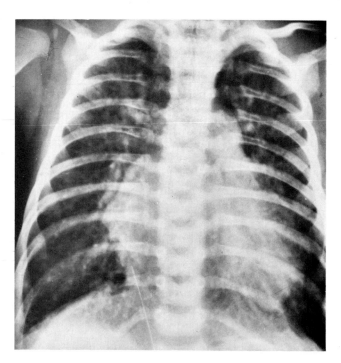

Left atrial enlargement, therefore, is not found in atrial septal defect and endocardial cushion defect; it is present in patients with ventricular septal defect or patent ductus arteriosus.

In patients with left atrial enlargement, the size of the aorta should be evaluated. This is frequently difficult in infants, since the great vessels may be obscured by the thymus. In patients with an extracardiac shunt, such as patent ductus arteriosus, the aorta and main pulmonary artery are of equal size (Fig. 5–1), while in an intracardiac shunt (e.g., ventricular septal defect), the aorta is inconspicuous compared to the enlarged main pulmonary artery (Fig. 5–2).

The cardiac anomalies in this category account for nearly half of all cases of congenital heart disease. The clinical, laboratory, and radiographic findings vary considerably, depending upon the hemodynamics. Those with large defects and greatly increased blood flow show a slow growth, develop frequent respiratory infections including pneumonia, and develop congestive cardiac failure.

Ventricular Septal Defect

Ventricular septal defect is the most common congenital cardiac anomaly. It is present as an isolated lesion in 20 per cent of patients with congenital heart disease and coexists with other anomalies such as patent ductus arteriosus or coarctation of the aorta in another 5 per cent of patients.

The ventricular septal defect can be located in various positions in the interventricular septum.

Since the subaortic area of the left ventricle passes obliquely behind the

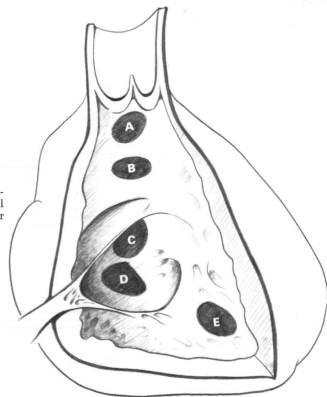

FIGURE 5–3. Location of ventricular septal defects. *A*, Supracristal defect; *B*, cristal defect; *C*, membranous defect; *D*, posterior defect; *E*, muscular defect.

infundibulum of the right ventricle, ventricular septal defects located immediately below the aortic valve may emerge at different sites in the right ventricle.

The most common ventricular septal defects (Fig. 5–3) are:

1. Membranous ventricular septal defect (80 per cent). This defect is located in the membranous septum and adjacent muscular septum. The defect lies below the crista supraventricularis.

2. Muscular ventricular septal defects (10 per cent). These defects, which may be isolated or multiple, occur anywhere in the muscular ventricular septum. They are hidden within the coarse trabeculations of the right ventricular septum.

3. Ventricular septal defect of atrioventricular canal type (5 per cent). This defect involves the posterior ventricular septum and extends beneath the tricuspid annulus.

4. Supracristal ventricular septal defect (5 per cent). Located immediately beneath the pulmonary valve, the upper border lies beneath the right coronary cusp of the aortic valve.

Multiple ventricular defects may occur. The size of the defect, which can vary considerably, is more important in determining the hemodynamics and clinical findings than the location of the defect.

Natural History. The natural history of a ventricular septal defect may follow one of three courses:

1. Development of pulmonary vascular disease from progressive medial hypertrophy and intimal proliferation in pulmonary arterioles. The pulmonary vascular resistance rises and may eventually exceed systemic vascular resistance, causing blood to shunt from right-to-left and leading to cyanosis. This is called Eisenmenger's syndrome.

2. Development of infundibular stenosis. Three per cent of patients with a large ventricular septal defect develop infundibular stenosis secondary to hypertrophied muscle bundles in the right ventricle. If infundibular stenosis is great enough, the patient becomes cyanotic and the hemodynamics resemble those of tetralogy of Fallot.

3. Spontaneous closure of the ventricular septal defect. In 10 per cent of patients with a large ventricular septal defect, and 50 per cent with either a small or moderate-sized ventricular septal defect, the defect spontaneously closes or becomes significantly smaller.

Hemodynamics. The hemodynamics of ventricular septal defect are determined by the size of the defect and the status of the pulmonary vasculature.

Ventricular septal defect may be broadly divided into two groups:

1. Large (Fig. 5–4). The size of the defect is at least 75 per cent of the size of the aorta. Left ventricular systolic pressure equals right ventricular systolic pressure, and relative pulmonary and systemic vascular resistances influence the magnitude of the shunt through the defect.

2. Small or medium-sized (Fig. 5–5). The size of the defect is less than 75 per cent the size of the aorta. Left ventricular systolic pressure exceeds the right ventricular systolic pressure. The size of the defect and the pressure difference across the defect determine the size of the left-to-right shunt.

Normally, pulmonary vascular resistance is elevated at birth and declines rapidly during early infancy. With the decrease of pulmonary vascular resistance, pulmonary blood flow increases significantly through the defect and lungs. The large volume of blood returning to the left atrium and left ventricle causes left ventricular dilatation. The volume load upon the left ventricle in the presence of a large ventricular septal defect may exceed the compensatory mechanism of

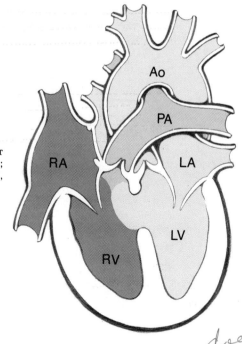

FIGURE 5–4. The central circulation with a large ventricular septal defect. Left-to-right shunt. Ao, Aorta; LA, left atrium; LV, left ventricle; PA, pulmonary artery; RA, right atrium; RV, right ventricle.

hypertrophy. Consequently, congestive cardiac failure typically develops at about two to three months of age.

In patients with a small or moderate-sized ventricular septal defect, pulmonary vascular resistance decreases normally, and usually the volume of pulmonary blood flow is limited by the size of the defect. Therefore, heart failure does not occur among these patients.

Clinical Features. The clinical findings vary considerably. The majority of

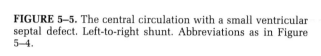

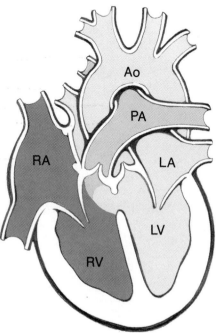

FIGURE 5–5. The central circulation with a small ventricular septal defect. Left-to-right shunt. Abbreviations as in Figure 5–4.

patients have small or moderate-sized ventricular septal defects and are therefore asymptomatic. Most patients with large ventricular septal defects develop congestive cardiac failure at two to three months of age.

The typical auscultatory finding is a loud pansystolic murmur, often associated with a thrill, heard best along the left sternal border. Additional findings include a loud P_2, if pulmonary hypertension is present, and an apical diastolic murmur from increased blood flow across the mitral valve, if the volume of pulmonary blood flow is at least twice normal.

Echocardiographic Features. The echocadiogram is most useful in patients with ventricular septal defect when identifying coexistent conditions such as atrial septal defect or obstructive lesions of either the left or the right ventricular outflow areas.

With the development of cross-sectional echocardiography, the location of the defect in the septum can usually be identified, and this provides useful information to surgeons (Fig. 5–6). Most ventricular septal defects greater than 4 mm in diameter can be identified by cross-sectional echocardiography—by a dropout of septal echoes in the presence of satisfactory echoes recorded from other portions of the ventricular septum. It is more difficult to identify a ventricular septal defect on M-mode echocardiograms.

Increased left atrial and left ventricular dimensions are present in patients with a considerable-sized left-to-right shunt. Increased right atrial dimension and wall thickness are present in patients with pulmonary hypertension.

Radiographic Features. Because of the variation in size and hemodynamics, the radiographic appearance of a ventricular septal defect is not uniform. In most patients a correct diagnosis can be made when clinical information is considered by the radiologist. The chest radiogram generally reflects the hemodynamics.

1. Small ventricular septal defects (small shunt and normal PA pressures).
    a. Cardiac size is normal.
    b. The pulmonary arterial segment and pulmonary vasculature appear normal.
    c. The left atrium is not enlarged, since the pulmonary blood flow is not large enough to distend the left atrium.
    d. A ventricular septal defect with a 2 to 1 shunt may be associated with minimal or borderline radiographic findings (Fig. 5–7).
2. Medium (50 per cent or more shunt) (Fig. 5–8).
    a. Cardiac size is slightly enlarged.
    b. The pulmonary arterial segment and vascularity are at the upper limits of normal or increased.
    c. The left atrium is enlarged.

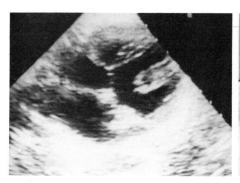 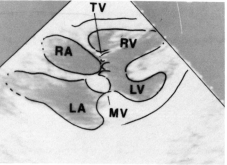

FIGURE 5–6. Cross-sectional echocardiogram. Subcostal view. Large membranous ventricular septal defect. Communication is present between left ventricle (LV) and right ventricle (RV).

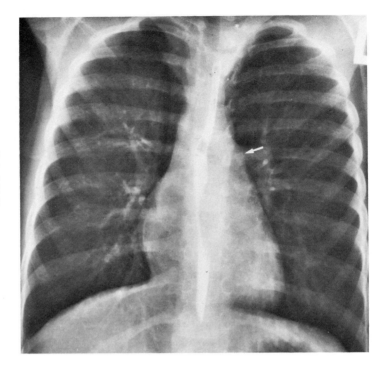

FIGURE 5–7. Small ventricular septal defect. Normal pulmonary arterial vascularity. Normal cardiac size. Slight prominence of the pulmonary artery segment (arrow).

3. Large ventricular septal defects (large pulmonary blood flow and pulmonary hypertension) (Fig. 5–9).
   a. The cardiac size is moderately or markedly enlarged (Fig. 5–9A), because the increased volume of pulmonary blood flow enlarges the left ventricle.
   b. The pulmonary arterial segment is enlarged. The pulmonary vasculature is markedly increased and has a fluffy appearance similar to atrial septal defect.

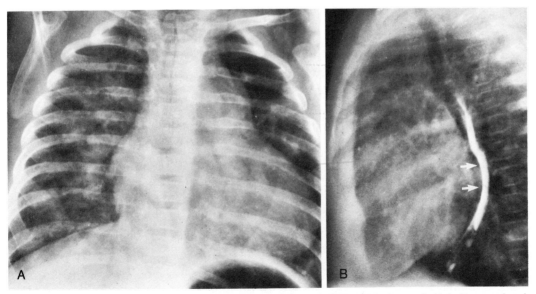

FIGURE 5–8. Moderate ventricular septal defect. *A*, Posteroanterior projection. Increased pulmonary arterial vascularity. Cardiomegaly. Prominent main pulmonary artery segment. *B*, Lateral projection. Fullness of retrosternal space produced by a large right ventricle. Left atrial enlargement causing displacement of the barium column (arrows).

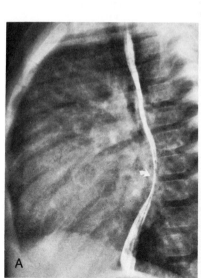 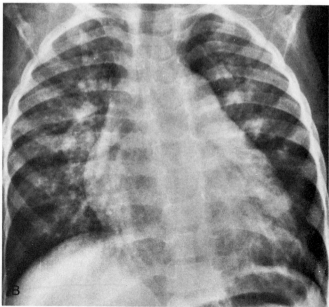

FIGURE 5–9. Large ventricular septal defect. *A*, Posteroanterior projection. Marked increased pulmonary arterial vascularity. Indistinct vascular markings. Cardiomegaly. Lateral displacement of cardiac apex. Prominent main pulmonary artery segment. *B*, Lateral projection. Left atrial enlargement (arrow). Right-sided cardiac enlargement evidenced by partial obliteration of the retrosternal space.

    c. Left atrial enlargement is evident on the left anterior oblique or lateral views (Fig. 5–9*B*). Enlargement of the left atrium reflects the volume of pulmonary blood flow.

    d. Right ventricular hypertrophy causes retrosternal fullness.

4. Ventricular septal defect with very high pulmonary vascular resistance. As pulmonary vascular resistance increases, the left-to-right shunt decreases. The following x-ray changes are noted (Fig. 5–10):

    a. Left atrial enlargement disappears.

    b. Cardiac size becomes smaller.

    c. The central pulmonary arteries become more enlarged and tortuous.

    d. The peripheral pulmonary arteries become constricted, producing the appearance of "pruning."

    e. Right ventricular hypertrophy causes fullness of the retrosternal space.

    f. Calcification may be observed in the main and large pulmonary arterial branches because of the atherosclerotic plaques that develop secondary to long-standing pulmonary hypertension.

    In patients with a ventricular septal defect, when the shunt decreases either from the defect undergoing closure or from the development of right ventricular outflow obstruction, cardiac size decreases, left atrial enlargement disappears, and pulmonary vasculature decreases, particularly in the peripheral lung fields.

    The radiographic differentiation among these three events, which lead to a reduction of pulmonary blood flow, is difficult. A ventricular septal defect without prominent pulmonary artery segment, however, suggests the presence of infundibular stenosis (pink tetrad) (Fig. 5–11). If a right aortic arch coexists with a left-to-right shunt, the most likely diagnosis is ventricular septal defect. When the right arch does not have an aortic diverticulum, pulmonary stenosis usually coexists.

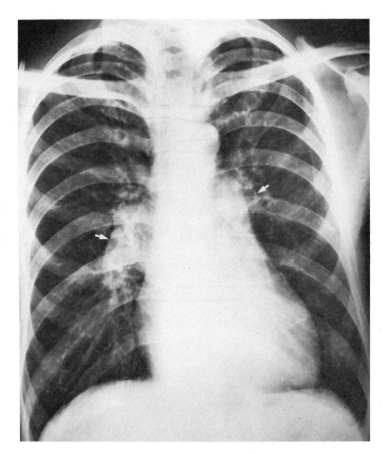

FIGURE 5–10. Ventricular septal defect with very high pulmonary vascular resistance. Large central hilar vessels. Linear calcifications (arrows) in the walls of the right and left pulmonary arteries. Rapid tapering of arteries toward the periphery. Cardiomegaly. Prominent main pulmonary artery segment.

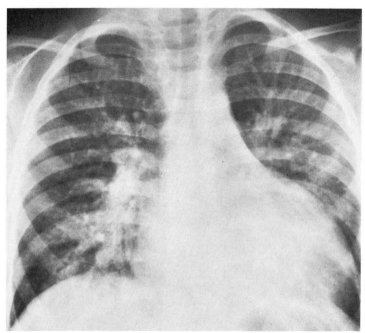

FIGURE 5–11. Infundibular stenosis. Increased pulmonary arterial vascularity. Large central hilar vessels. Cardiomegaly. Lateral displacement of cardiac apex. Concave pulmonary artery segment.

Some patients with a large ventricular septal defect are treated by pulmonary artery banding to reduce the size of the left-to-right shunt. Similar radiographic changes will develop, as in patients with other causes, decreasing the volume of left-to-right shunt. If the pulmonary artery band is properly placed, the pulmonary blood flow decreases equally in both lung fields. Chest films should be examined carefully to detect a unilateral decrease of pulmonary flow. Such a finding suggests migration of the band and consequent compression of one of the pulmonary arteries. Compression of the right pulmonary artery occurs more commonly (Fig. 5–12).

Angiographic Appearance. In ventricular septal defect, left ventriculography is needed to determine the number and location of the defects in order to provide information to the surgeon. Right ventriculography and aortography are indicated in patients with elevated right ventricular systolic pressure in order to exclude a major coexistent cardiac anomaly.

Because of the crescent-shape of the ventricular septum, and its position and orientation within the thorax, left ventriculography using axial projections (Fig. 5–13) is indispensable for precise angiographic evaluation of ventricular septal defect. Several projections are needed to demonstrate the various types of ventricular septal defect:

1. Membranous ventricular septal defects are best demonstrated by the horizontal plane of the long-axial oblique view (Fig. 5–13).

2. Muscular ventricular septal defects, either isolated or multiple, are best demonstrated by horizontal plane of a long-axial oblique projection (Fig. 5–14). Different degrees of obliquity may be needed to demonstrate the defect on profile.

3. Ventricular septal defects, lying posteriorly beneath the tricuspid valve (atrioventricular canal type), are best demonstrated by the vertical x-ray tube using a hepatoclavicular projection.

4. A supracristal ventricular septal defect is best demonstrated by the vertical

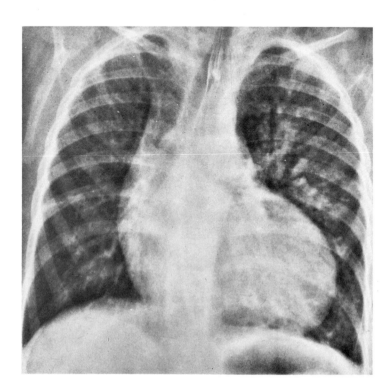

FIGURE 5–12. Compression of the right pulmonary artery. Asymmetrical pulmonary arterial markings, diminished in the right lung field. Cardiomegaly. Round, slightly uptilted apex.

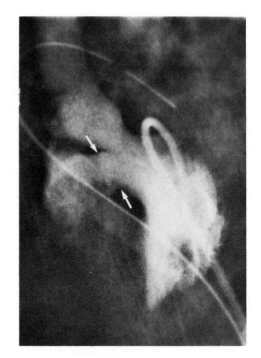

FIGURE 5–13. Large membranous ventricular septal defect (white arrows). Left ventriculogram in long-axial oblique projection.

x-ray tube using a long axial oblique projection (Fig. 5–15) or a straight lateral projection (Fig. 5–16). Following a left ventriculogram, opacification of the right ventricular outflow tract and pulmonary artery typically occurs.

Management. The management of ventricular septal defects varies according to the age of the patient, the size of the ventricular septal defect, and the hemodynamics.

Approximately 10 per cent of ventricular septal defects are large and cause cardiac failure at about three months of age. These infants are treated with digitalis and diuretics. If, after treatment, findings of cardiac failure persist, operative treatment is indicated. The type of operation varies among surgeons. There are two options: (1) banding of the pulmonary artery with a strip of Dacron

FIGURE 5–14. Large ventricular septal defect (arrows) in muscular septum. Left ventriculogram in long-axial oblique projection.

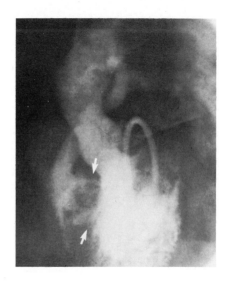

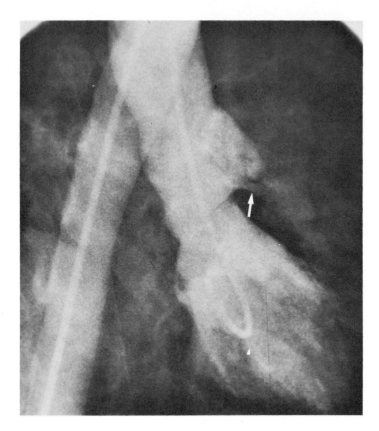

FIGURE 5–15. Supracristal ventricular septal defect. Left ventriculogram in long-axial oblique projection. Vertical plane. Jet of contrast medium (white arrow) from left ventricle directly into subpulmonic area. Crista supraventricularis below ventricular septal defect.

to narrow the pulmonary arterial lumen, thereby reducing the volume of pulmonary blood flow. This procedure, if used, is applied to very small infants or to infants with muscular or multiple ventricular septal defects; (2) correction of the ventricular septal defect with a patch.

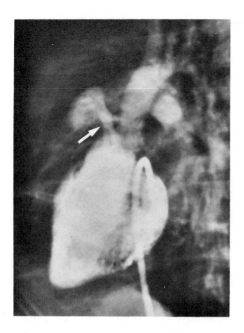

FIGURE 5–16. Supracristal ventricular septal defect. Left ventriculogram in lateral projection. Narrow jet of contrast medium (arrow) from left ventricle into subpulmonic area.

If the infant responds to treatment of congestive heart failure, an operation to close the ventricular defect is delayed until about 18 months of age. The mortality rate is low at this age, and the chance of developing pulmonary vascular disease is remote.

Among 90 per cent who are asymptomatic, those with clinical or catheterization evidence of a large shunt or elevated pulmonary arterial pressure, the ventricular septal defect is closed operatively at 18 months of age. Otherwise, if there is clinical evidence that the shunt is not large or pulmonary arterial pressure is not elevated, the patient is followed. In many of these patients the ventricular septal defect tends to become smaller or to close spontaneously.

Selected Bibliography

Capelli, H., Andrade, J. L., and Somerville, J.: Classification of the site of ventricular septal defect by 2-dimensional echocardiography. Am. J. Cardiol., 51:1474–1480, 1983.

Fellows, K. E., Westerman, G. R., and Keane, J. F.: Angiocardiography of multiple ventricular septal defects in infancy. Circulation, 66(5):1094–1099, 1982.

Goor, D. A., Lillehei, W., Rees, R., and Edwards, J. E.: Isolated ventricular septal defect: Development basis for various types and presentation of classification. Chest, 58:468–482, 1970.

Otterstad, J. E., Nitter-Hauge, S., and Myhre, E.: Isolated ventricular septal defect in adults: Clinical and haemodynamic findings. Br. Heart J., 50:343–348, 1983.

Patent Ductus Arteriosus

Patent ductus arteriosus represents 8 to 10 per cent of all instances of congenital heart disease. It occurs twice as frequently in females as in males. The incidence is considerably higher among prematurely born infants, particularly those with the respiratory distress syndrome.

Anatomic Features. Patent ductus arteriosus connects the left pulmonary artery with the descending aorta immediately beyond the origin of the left subclavian artery. Patent ductus arteriosus is a normal pathway of the fetal circulation, allowing blood to flow from the pulmonary artery into the descending aorta. Normally, the ductus arteriosus closes functionally by 48 hours of age and, anatomically, by one month of age. When the ductus arteriosus fails to close, a communication persists between the two great vessels and allows a shunt from aorta to pulmonary artery.

Hemodynamics. The ductus can vary in length and caliber. A long or narrow ductus allows a small shunt because of the high resistance to flow. A wide ductus allows a large volume of left-to-right shunt and in these there is equalization of aortic and pulmonary arterial pressures, and pulmonary hypertension (Fig. 5–17).

The direction and magnitude of flow through a large patent ductus arteriosus depends on the relative resistances of the pulmonary and systemic vascular beds. Since pulmonary vascular resistance normally is less than systemic vascular resistance, blood flows from left to right through the ductus. Flow occurs from right to left through the ductus when the pulmonary vascular resistance is elevated or the resistance is low in the descending aorta, occurring from a high degree of obstruction on the left side of the heart, as in conditions such as aortic atresia, interruption of the aortic arch, or severe coarctation of the aorta.

Clinical Features. Other than prematurely born infants, most patients with patent ductus arteriosus are asymptomatic. In the few with a large left-to-right shunt, congestive cardiac failure usually develops by the age of three months. Patent ductus arteriosus is usually ascertained by the discovery of a continuous murmur. The typical continuous murmur of a patent ductus arteriosus may be found in a neonate, and in some neonates the murmur disappears spontaneously. More commonly, the murmur is found on subsequent examination during infancy.

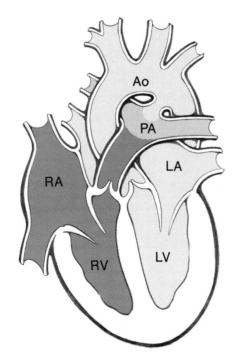

FIGURE 5–17. The central circulation with a large patent ductus arteriosus. Left-to-right shunt. Ao, Aorta; LA, left atrium; LV, left ventricle; PA, pulmonary artery; RA, right atrium; RV, right ventricle.

Echocardiographic Features. M-mode echocardiograms are used to assess the hemodynamics of patent ductus arteriosus by measuring left atrial or left ventricular dimensions. Changes in these dimensions are used to follow serially the course of the ductus in premature infants, but these dimensions correlate only roughly with hemodynamics.

On two-dimensional echocardiograms, a moderate or large-sized patent ductus arteriosus can be identified as a tubular arching structure located between the proximal left pulmonary artery and descending aorta (Fig. 5–18). It is best viewed in a suprasternal projection.

Radiographic Features. The radiographic findings are not uniform, but a correct diagnosis can usually be made when clinical findings are considered.

The radiographic features vary with the hemodynamics.

1. Small patent ductus arteriosus (small shunt and normal pulmonary arterial pressure).
   a. Cardiac size is normal.

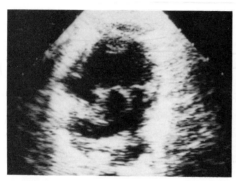
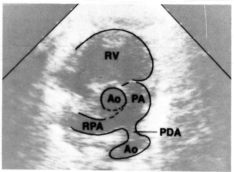

FIGURE 5–18. Patent ductus arteriosus (PDA). Cross-sectional echocardiogram. Ao, aorta; RV, right ventricle; PA, pulmonary artery; RPA, right pulmonary artery.

    b. Pulmonary arterial segment and pulmonary vasculature are normal.

    c. Left atrium is not enlarged, since the volume of pulmonary blood flow is not large enough to distend the left atrium.

    d. A patent ductus arteriosus with a 2 to 1 shunt may be associated with minimal or borderline radiographic findings.

2. Moderate-sized patent ductus arteriosus (50 per cent shunt and normal or moderate elevation of pulmonary artery pressure) (Fig. 5–19A).

    a. Cardiac size is normal.

    b. Pulmonary arterial segment and pulmonary vascularity are at the upper limits of normal or increased.

    c. Left atrial enlargement is present

3. Large patent ductus arteriosus (large pulmonary blood flow and pulmonary hypertension) (Fig. 5–19B).

    a. Cardiac size is moderately or markedly enlarged, because of an increased left ventricular volume secondary to the increased pulmonary blood flow.

    b. The pulmonary arterial segment is enlarged. The pulmonary vasculature is markedly increased and has a "fluffy" appearance.

    c. Left atrial enlargement is present.

    d. Right ventricular hypertrophy occurring from increased pulmonary artery pressure causes retrosternal fullness.

    e. The ascending aorta and aortic arch are enlarged. —key

4. Large patent ductus arteriosus with severe pulmonary vascular disease. Pulmonary blood flow is limited.

    a. Left atrial enlargement disappears.

    b. Cardiac size becomes smaller.

    c. Pulmonary trunk and central pulmonary arteries remain enlarged and the latter remains tortuous.

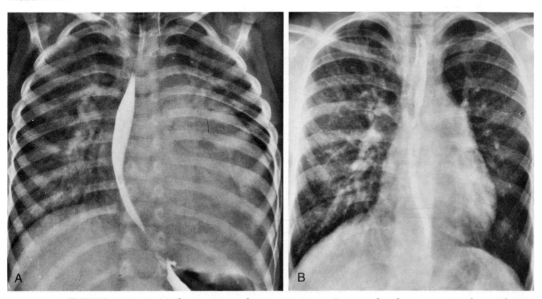

FIGURE 5–19. A, Moderate patent ductus arteriosus. Increased pulmonary arterial vascularity, more prominent on the right side. Normal cardiac size. Prominent main pulmonary artery segment. Slight left atrial enlargement (displacement of the esophagus toward the right side). B, Large patent ductus arteriosus. Markedly increased pulmonary arterial vascularity. Haziness of vascular markings from interstitial congestion. Marked cardiomegaly. Left atrial enlargement (displacement of the barium-filled esophagus toward the right). Prominent main pulmonary artery segment.

    d. Peripheral pulmonary arteries become constricted.

    e. Calcifications may be observed in pulmonary trunk or major pulmonary arteries.

    f. Right ventricular hypertrophy causes retrosternal fullness.

These radiographic features mimic ventricular septal defect, but there are specific additional features that suggest patent ductus arteriosus.

1. Pulmonary blood flow may be unequally distributed with less blood flow occurring to the left lung, particularly the left upper lobe (Fig. 5–20).

2. The ascending aorta and aortic arch to the level of the ductus are enlarged in patients with a large shunt (Fig. 5–20). An enlarged thymus may obscure this finding radiographically.

3. In some infants, a patent ductus arteriosus may be seen either as a faint linear density visible through the pulmonary artery or as a prominence between the aortic knob and pulmonary arterial segment along the upper left cardiac border.

4. The ductus, either ligamentous or patent, may calcify. Calcification in the form of a ring suggests patency.

Angiographic Appearance. Usually the diagnosis of patent ductus arteriosus is made on the basis of auscultatory findings. Occasionally angiography is needed to make the diagnosis (Fig. 5–21). Aortography with injection of contrast material into the aortic arch is the procedure of choice in the evaluation of a patent ductus arteriosus. Balloon occlusion aortography produces an excellent demonstration (Fig. 5–22). The ductus arteriosus is best visualized in the lateral or left anterior oblique projection. It arches anteriorly from the anterior wall of the aorta to the

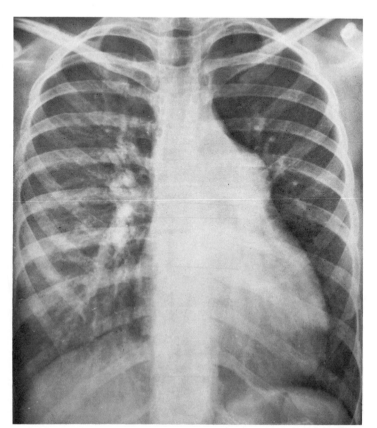

FIGURE 5–20. Patent ductus arteriosus. Asymmetry of vascular markings, more increased in the right lung. Mild cardiomegaly, with a left ventricular configuration. Prominent pulmonary artery segment. Left aortic knob.

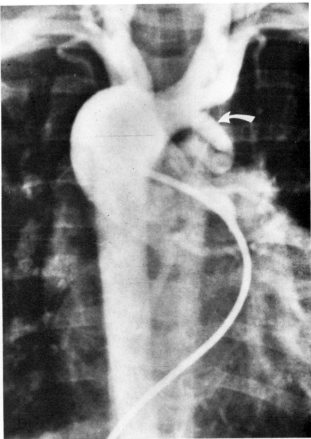

FIGURE 5–21. Patent ductus arteriosus. A, Aortogram. Lateral projection. Patent ductus arteriosus. B, Catheter advanced from the inferior vena cava through the right ventricle and ventricular septal defect into the ascending aorta. Right aortic arch. Large tortuous patent ductus arteriosus connects with pulmonary artery (arrow).

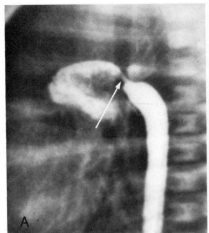

proximal part of the left pulmonary artery. Its course parallels the aortic arch. The aortic end of the ductus is often wide (ductus diverticulum), and it often tapers toward its connection with the left pulmonary artery.

   Management. In all patients, a patent ductus arteriosus with a left-to-right shunt should be closed. In most patients this is accomplished by ligating and

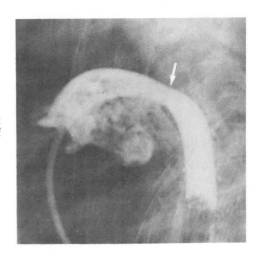

FIGURE 5–22. Balloon occlusion aortogram. Large patent ductus arteriosus (arrow) in patient with interruption of the aortic arch.

dividing the ductus through a left thoracotomy, usually at the time the ductus is discovered. Generally, cardiac catheterization and angiography are not necessary to establish a diagnosis of patent ductus arteriosus or to prepare the patient for operation.

A patent ductus arteriosus occurring in a premature infant may be managed differently, although we still prefer operation for this group, as well. In premature infants, indomethacin has been administered in an attempt to close the ductus, because this drug blocks the synthesis of prostaglandins. Prostaglandin E_1 is a potent dilator of the ductus. Medical management is associated with closure or minution of the size of the ductus in perhaps two thirds of infant patients.

Selected Bibliography

The Ductus Arteriosus. Report of the 75th Ross Conference on Pediatric Research. Henmann, M. A., and Rudolph, A. M. (Eds.). Ross Laboratories, Columbus, Ohio 43216 (publishers).

Margulis, A. R., Figley, M. M., and Stern, A. M.: Unusual roentgen manifestations of patent ductus arteriosus. Radiology, *63*(3):334–345, 1954.

Rudolph, A. M., Mayer, F. E., Nadas, A. S., and Gross, R. E.: Patent ductus arteriosus: A clinical hemodynamic study of 23 patients in the first year of life. Pediatrics, *22*:892–904, 1958.

Smallhorn, J. F., Huhta, J. C., Anderson, R. H., and Macartney, F. J.: Suprasternal cross-sectional echocardiography in assessment of patent ductus arteriosus. Br. Heart J., *48*:321–330, 1982.

Other Conditions with Left Atrial Enlargement
— anything listed — to mitral valve

Several uncommon conditions also account for increased pulmonary arterial markings and left atrial enlargement.

1. Aorticopulmonary window. This is a communication, usually large, between the ascending aorta and main pulmonary artery. The hemodynamics and clinical picture resemble a large patent ductus arteriosus. On the thoracic roentgenogram, however, the ascending aorta and arch are small, and the plain film findings mimic ventricular septal defect (Figs. 5–23 and 5–24).

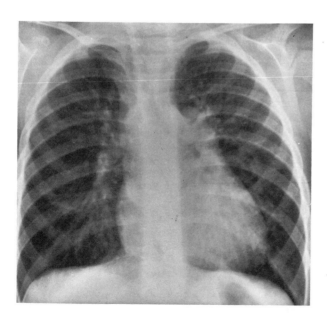

FIGURE 5–23. Aorticopulmonary window. Increased pulmonary arterial vascularity. Cardiomegaly. Prominent main pulmonary artery segment. Small aortic knob.

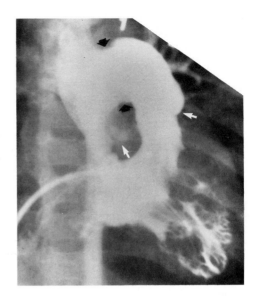

FIGURE 5–24. Right ventriculogram in anteroposterior projection. Large communication between pulmonary artery and ascending aorta (black arrows). Separate semilunar valves (white arrows).

2. Ruptured sinus of Valsalva aneurysm. An aneurysm of the sinus of Valsalva may rupture into the right atrium or right ventricle and lead to a left-to-right shunt from the aorta. Rupture can also occur into the left ventricle and left atrium. The dilated right- or left-sided cardiac chambers are evident radiographically (Figs. 5–25 and 5–26). The diagnosis is usually confirmed by characteristic continuous murmurs along lower left or right sternal borders.

3. Coronary arteriovenous fistula. These fistulae, which may occur between either small or large branches of coronary arteries and veins, are usually small and do not cause radiographic changes. They are diagnosed by recognition of typical continuous murmurs (Fig. 5–27).

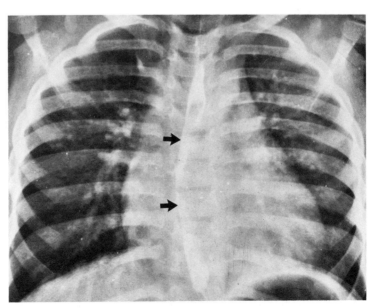

FIGURE 5–25. Ruptured sinus of Valsalva aneurysm into the right ventricle. Increased pulmonary arterial vascularity. Cardiomegaly. Slight displacement of barium column (arrows) to the right by enlarged left atrium.

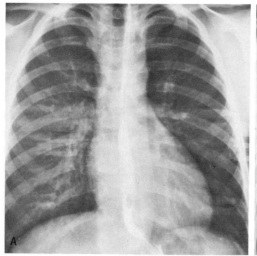

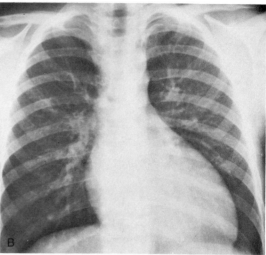

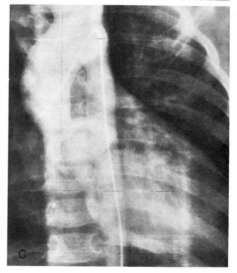

FIGURE 5–26. Ruptured sinus of Valsalva aneurysm into the left ventricle. *A,* Before rupture. Normal pulmonary arterial vascularity. Normal cardiac size. *B,* Following rupture. Normal pulmonary arterial vascularity. Cardiomegaly. Left ventricular configuration. *C,* Aortogram. Anteroposterior projection. Domed aortic valve. Deformed left sinus of Valsalva. Massive aortic insufficiency.

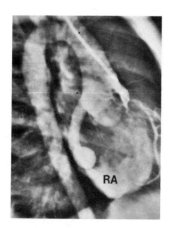

FIGURE 5–27. Coronary arteriovenous fistula. Aortogram. Markedly dilated circumflex coronary artery connecting to the right atrium (RA).

Selected Bibliography

Neufeld, H. N., Lester, R. G. Adams, P., Anderson, R. C., Lillehei, C. W., and Edwards, J. E.: Aorticopulmonary septal defect. Am. J. Cardiol., *9*(1):12–25, 1962.

Atrial Septal Defect

Atrial septal defect is the fifth (8 per cent) most common form of congenital heart disease and is the most common type of congenital heart disease in adults, since the life span in unoperated cases may be 50 years.

Anatomy. Most atrial septal defects are large and allow free communication between the left and right atria.

Six anatomic types of atrial septal defects exist (Fig. 5–28):

1. Sinus venosus atrial septal defect. This defect is located above the fossa ovalis and adjacent to the entrance to the superior vena cava. It is frequently associated with anomalous drainage of the right pulmonary veins.

2. Atrial septal defect of the ostium secundum type. This, the most common type of defect, is located in the region of the fossa ovalis.

3. Defect at the junction of the inferior vena cava and the right atrium.

4. Defect posterior to fossa ovalis.

5. Atrial septal defect in the region of the coronary sinus. This defect is associated with the connection of the persistent left superior vena cava to the left atrium and absent coronary sinus.

6. Ostium primum atrial septal defect. This defect, located in the lowermost part of the atrial septum, is part of the spectrum of endocardial cushion defect and will be discussed in the following section.

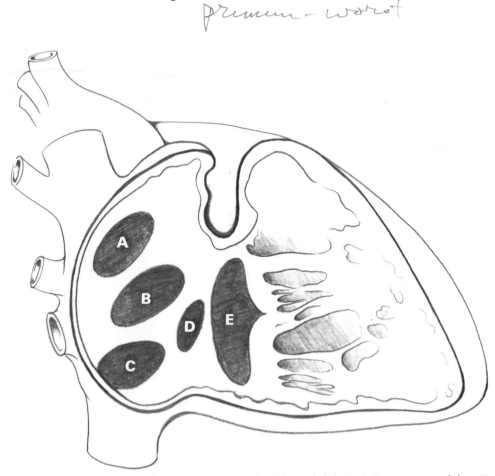

FIGURE 5–28. Location of the common types of atrial septal defects. *A*, Sinus venosus defect; *B*, ostium secundum defect; *C*, inferior vena cava defect; *D*, defect at site of coronary sinus; *E*, ostium primum defect.

Hemodynamics. In most instances a left-to-right shunt occurs through the atrial septal defect and results in an increased volume of blood circulating through the right side of the heart (Fig. 5–29). Enlargement of the right atrium, right ventricle, and pulmonary artery results. The right ventricle is not hypertrophied unless pulmonary hypertension develops. The left ventricle may be slightly smaller than normal. The left atrium is not enlarged even though a larger than normal volume of blood passes through it, since it can empty easily through the atrial septal defect into the right atrium.

Since the defect is large, atrial pressures are equal. Therefore, ventricular distensibility or compliance is the major factor governing the direction and size of the left-to-right shunt. The right ventricular wall is thinner than the left ventricular wall, and therefore the right ventricle is more compliant or distensible. At equal atrial pressures, more blood flows into the right ventricle than into the left. In most patients with atrial septal defect, the size of the left-to-right shunt is about 3 to 1. The systemic cardiac output is normal at rest.

With each decade after the third, the incidence of pulmonary vascular disease increases among patients with atrial septal defect. With the elevation of pulmonary arterial pressure, right ventricular hypertrophy develops, right ventricular compliance drops, and the shunt may eventually become right-to-left.

Clinical Features. In contrast to conditions with a left-to-right shunt at either the ventricular or the great vessel level, patients with large atrial septal defects do not usually develop symptoms, since the left-to-right shunts occur at a low pressure. These shunts may be tolerated for decades before decompensation occurs. Auscultatory findings are diagnostic, and are caused by the increased blood flow across the pulmonary and tricuspid valves. There is pulmonary systolic ejection murmur, tricuspid diastolic murmur, and wide, fixed splitting of S_2.

The electrocardiogram in most patients shows mild right axis deviation and an rSR' pattern, frequently called an incomplete right bundle-branch block

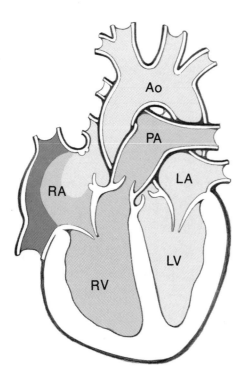

FIGURE 5–29. The central circulation in atrial septal defect. Left-to-right shunt. Ao, Aorta; LA, left atrium; LV, left ventricle; PA, pulmonary artery; RA, right atrium; RV, right ventricle.

pattern, which reflects the increased right ventricular volume. Right atrial enlargement is found in half of the patients.

Echocardiographic Features. The M-mode echocardiogram supports the hemodynamic pattern by reflecting the increased right ventricular volume. The right ventricular internal dimension is increased. Paradoxical septal motion is found, indicating that the interventricular septum moves anteriorly (not posteriorly) during systole.

In cross-sectional echocardiography, the interatrial septum can be visualized on a subcostal view (Fig. 5–30). The drop-out of echoes is highly suggestive of a diagnosis of an atrial septal defect. The location of the defect, but not its size, can be determined echocardiographically.

Radiographic Features. The radiographic findings vary. Some patients with a large left-to-right shunt may have a completely normal thoracic roentgenogram.

In most cases the radiographic findings are the following:

1. Increased pulmonary vascular markings. The markings may be indistinct, since pulmonary hypertension is not usually present. The central and peripheral pulmonary arteries are enlarged (Fig. 5–31A).
2. No left atrial enlargement. This finding helps to distinguish atrial septal defect from ventricular septal defect, patent ductus arteriosus, and other shunts at the ventricular or great vessel level (Fig. 5–31B).
3. Cardiomegaly from right atrial and right ventricular enlargement.
   a. Right atrial enlargement is evident on the posteroanterior view (Fig. 5–32).
   b. Right ventricular enlargement causes a fullness of retrosternal space or bulging of the sternum (Fig. 5–31B).
4. The cardiac contour may mimic left ventricular enlargement, since with clockwise rotation of the heart, the right ventricle forms the left cardiac border. The cardiac apex is, however, elevated (Fig. 5–31A).
5. Aortic knob might appear small. Since cardiac output is normal, the aorta is of normal size but is obscured by pulmonary trunk and clockwise rotation of the heart (Fig. 5–32).

Angiographic Appearance. In most cases cardiac catheterization and angiography are unnecessary to diagnose atrial septal defect, because the clinical features are so typical. During cardiac catheterization, indirect diagnosis of an atrial septal defect can be obtained during the late phase of a right ventriculogram, or of a pulmonary arteriogram, by observing the pulmonary venous return.

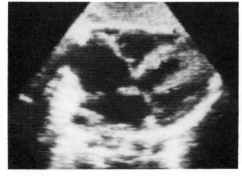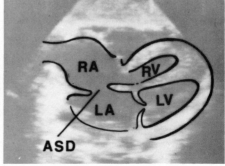

FIGURE 5–30. Atrial septal defect (ASD) of ostium secundum type. Cross-sectional echocardiogram, subcostal view. There is absence of echoes in the atrial septum, thus allowing communication between left and right atria. RA, Right atrium; LA, left atrium; RV, right ventricle; LV, left ventricle.

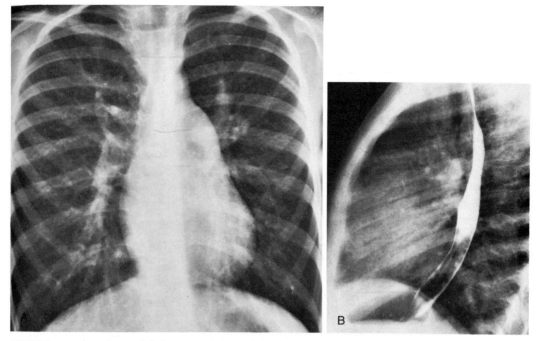

FIGURE 5–31. Atrial septal defect. *A*, Posteroanterior projection. Increased pulmonary arterial vascularity. Normal cardiac size. Uptilted cardiac apex. Prominent main pulmonary artery segment. *B*, Lateral projection. No left atrial enlargement. Fullness of the retrosternal space from right-sided cardiac enlargement.

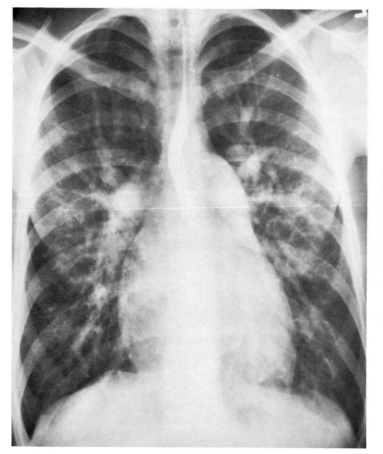

FIGURE 5–32. Atrial septal defect. Markedly increased pulmonary arterial vascularity. Enlarged hilar pulmonary arteries. Mild cardiomegaly. Prominent right heart border suggesting right atrial enlargement. Large pulmonary artery segment and small aortic knob suggests intracardiac shunt.

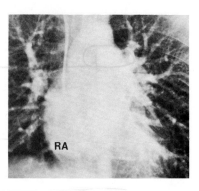

FIGURE 5–33. Atrial septal defect. Late phase of right ventriculogram in anteroposterior projection. Connection of pulmonary veins to left atrium. Contrast medium passes from left atrium to right atrium (RA).

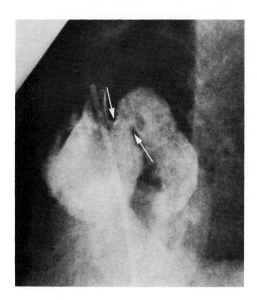

FIGURE 5–34. Atrial septal defect in tricuspid atresia. Right atriogram in hepatoclavicular view. Size and location of atrial septal defect are evident (arrows).

Following left atrial opacification, contrast medium shunts from the left atrium into the right atrium across the atrial septum (Fig. 5–33). A more direct angiographic demonstration of an atrial septal defect is obtained by injection of contrast material into the upper right pulmonary vein and obtaining films with the patient in an hepatoclavicular projection. In this projection the atrial septum is in profile, and the size and location of the atrial septal defect can be determined (Fig. 5–34).

Management. Atrial septal defects that are evident clinically should be closed by an operation, to either patch or suture the defect closed. The operation is usually performed in early childhood; the risk of operation is essentially zero.

Selected Bibliography

Gault, J. H., Morrow, A. G., Gay, W. A., Jr., and Ross, J., Jr.: Atrial septal defect in patients over the age of forty years: Clinical and hemodynamic studies and the effects of operation. Circulation, 38:261–272, 1968.

Shub, C., Dimopoulos, I. N., Seward, J. B., Callahan, J. A., Tancredi, R. G., Schattenberg, T. T., Reeder, G. S., Hagler, D. J., and Tajik, A. J.: Sensitivity to two-dimensional echocardiography in the direct visualization of atrial septal defect utilizing the subcostal approach: Experience with 154 patients. J. Am. Coll. Cardiol. 2(1):127–135, 1983.

Tandon, R., and Edwards, J. E.: Clinicopathologic correlations. Atrial septal defect in infancy: Common association with other anomalies. Circulation, 49:1005–1010, 1974.

Endocardial Cushion Defects

Abnormalities in the development of the endocardial cushion result in a broad spectrum of cardiac manifestations, which range from an isolated cleft in an atrioventricular valve to a complex anomaly that includes an ostium primum type atrial septal defect, ventricular septal defect, and tricuspid and mitral valve insufficiency. Endocardial cushion defects represent 4 to 5 per cent of instances of congenital heart disease and are the most common cardiac anomalies found in patients with Down's syndrome.

Embryology and Anatomy. Endocardial cushion tissue contributes to the formation of the ventricular septum, the lower part of the atrial septum, and the septal leaflets of the mitral and tricuspid valves (Chapter 1). If development of the endocardial cushions is arrested or interrupted, these portions of the heart do not develop properly.

Depending upon the timing of maldevelopment of the endocardial cushion tissue, three principal types of endocardial cushion defects exist:

1. Partial atrioventricular canal (Fig. 5–35). In this form, an ostium primum atrial septal defect is located low in the atrial septum immediately above the atrioventricular valvular annulus. A cleft in the septal leaflet of the mitral valve coexists, and occasionally there is a cleft in the tricuspid valve as well. The hemodynamics are those of an atrial level shunt and mitral regurgitation.

2. Transitional atrioventricular canal (Fig. 5–36). An atrial septal defect of the ostium primum type is present and continuous with a ventricular septal defect located immediately below the atrioventricular annulus. Clefts are present in the septal leaflets of both A-V valves. Because of the close attachment of the septal leaflets to the crest of the interventricular septal defect, a shunt does not occur at the ventricular level. The main hemodynamic abnormalities are mitral regurgitation and a left-to-right shunt at the atrial level.

3. Complete atrioventricular canal (Fig. 5–37). This less common anomaly involves the lower atrial septum and the adjacent portion of the ventricular septum. The clefts in the septal leaflets of the mitral and tricuspid valves are so complete that the atrioventricular valve leaflets are continuous across the ventricular septum and form two common atrioventricular leaflets, which extend from one ventricle to the other. The midportion of these leaflets is attached to the crest

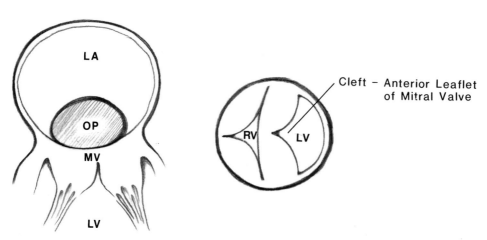

FIGURE 5–35. Partial atrioventricular canal. LA, left atrium; OP, ostum primum; MV, mitral valve; LA, left ventricle; RV, right ventricle; LV, left venricle.

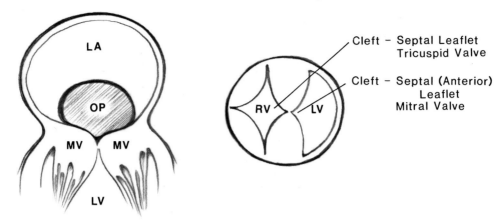

FIGURE 5–36. Transitional atrioventricular canal. LA, left atrium; OP, ostium primum; MV, mitral valve; LV, left ventricle; RV, right ventricle; LV, left ventricle.

of the ventricular septum, but a ventricular communication exists below these leaflets. There is associated pulmonary hypertension.

Clinical Features. Patients with complete atrioventricular canal become symptomatic in infancy, whereas patients with partial atrioventricular canal have few symptoms unless mitral insufficiency is severe. Characteristically, the infant with a complete endocardial cushion defect comes to attention because of poor weight gain, recurrent respiratory infections, and congestive heart failure.

Patients with complete atrioventricular canal have a tendency to develop pulmonary vascular disease early in life, with repeated pulmonary infections. Depending upon the hemodynamics, the auscultatory findings may be those of an atrial septal defect, ventricular septal defect, mitral regurgitation, or pulmonary hypertension. The electrocardiogram is diagnostic and shows left-axis deviation and incomplete right bundle-branch block. Biventricular hypertrophy may be present as well.

Hemodynamics. The hemodynamic manifestations depend upon the anatomic form and severity of the particular endocardiac cushion defect. In partial atrioventricular canal, the hemodynamics are those of an atrial septal defect and mitral

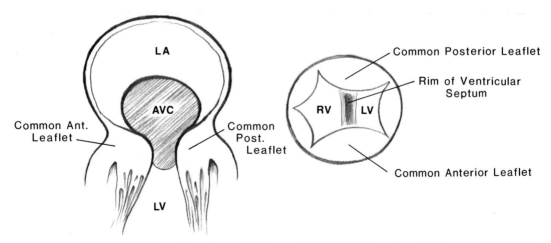

FIGURE 5–37. Complete atrioventricular canal (AVC). LA, left atrium; LV, left ventricle; RV, right ventricle; LV, left ventricle.

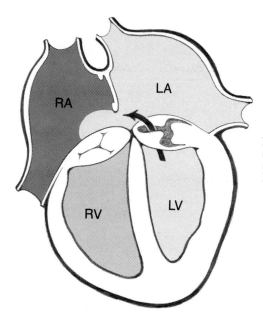

FIGURE 5–38. The central circulation in ostium primum atrial septal defect and cleft mitral valve. Left-to-right shunt. LA, left atrium; LV, left ventricle; RA, right atrium; RV, right ventricle.

regurgitation and depend upon the size of the atrial septal defect and degree of malfunction of the mitral valve (Fig. 5–38). In the transitional form, the atrial septal defect is usually large. The degree of mitral regurgitation varies considerably among patients. If the atrial septal defect is large, the effects of mitral valve incompetence are transmitted mainly to the right side of the heart, since the left atrium decompresses easily through the atrial septal defect. If the atrial septal defect is small, however, the left atrium and ventricle enlarge proportionally to the amount of mitral regurgitation, since they cannot decompress into the right side of the heart.

In complete endocardial cushion defect, the cardiac chambers are in free communication and left-to-right shunts occur at both the atrial and ventricular levels (Fig. 5–39). Because the right ventricle is more compliant, the left-to-right

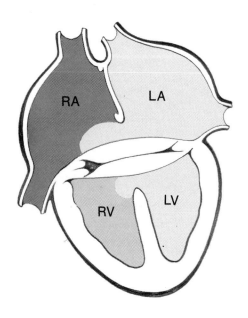

FIGURE 5–39. The central circulation in the presence of a complete atrioventricular canal. Common atrioventricular valve. Ventricular component. Left-to-right shunt. Abbreviations as in Figure 5–38.

atrial shunt places volume overload on the right atrium, right ventricle, and pulmonary artery. Each becomes dilated. The ventricular communication is usually large and is a major factor in determining the level of the pulmonary arterial pressure. The incidence of pulmonary hypertension in complete endocardial cushion defects is higher than that of partial atrioventricular canal without a ventricular septal defect. Pulmonary vascular disease can develop, and when severe, causes the shunt to become right to left. Either atrioventricular valve, but usually the mitral valve, can be insufficient. The severity of mitral regurgitation varies greatly.

Echocardiographic Features. Both the M-mode and two-dimensional echocardiograms are diagnostic. On M-mode echo, the following features suggest an ostium primum defect: increased internal dimension of the right ventricle and paradoxical septal motion, both of which are features of the atrial septal defect. In addition, the appearance of the anterior mitral valve leaflet is abnormal. During systole there may be multiple echoes, and during diastole this leaflet approaches the interventricular septum or may appear to cross the plane of the interventricular septum immediately above the atrioventricular annulus. The cleft in the anterior leaflet may be visualized.

In patients with complete atrioventricular canal, M-mode echocardiograms show little or no apparent interventricular septum, and absence of interventricular septum separating the mitral and tricuspid valves, so that during diastole the leaflets appear continuous across the plane of the septum. Cross-sectional echocardiography, using a subcostal and short-axis projection, shows the extent of the defect in the septa (Figs. 5–40 and 5–41).

Radiographic Features. The diagnosis of endocardial cushion defect can usually be made radiographically, particularly when clinical information, especially the finding of left-axis deviation on the electrocardiogram, is available.

The common radiographic features are (1) Lack of left atrial enlargement in the presence of increased pulmonary vascular markings. This finding indicates an atrial level shunt (Fig. 5–42A). (2) Enlargement of the cardiac contour out of proportion to the pulmonary vascularity. In endocardial cushion defect, unlike most other common forms of congenital heart disease, two factors, the left-to-right shunt and mitral regurgitation, contribute to dilatation of the heart and produce cardiomegaly (Fig. 5–42B).

In patients with partial or transitional atrioventricular canal, the thoracic

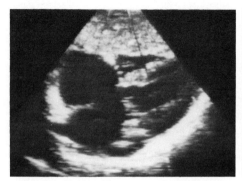
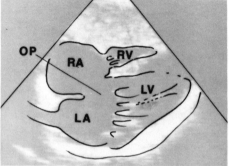

FIGURE 5–40. Complete atrioventricular canal. Cross-sectional echocardiogram, subcostal four-chamber view. Ostium primum defect (OP) is evidenced as a deficiency in the echoes of the atrial septum located immediately above the ventricles. RA, Right atrium; LA, left atrium; RV, right ventricle; LV, left ventricle.

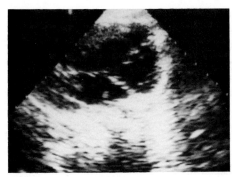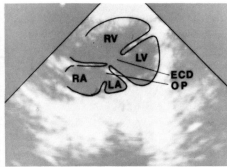

FIGURE 5–41. Complete endocardial cushion defect. Cross-sectional echocardiogram, apical subcostal view. There is a ventricular communication (ECD) and ostium primum (OP) defect, located below and above the level of atrioventricular valves, respectively. RA, right atrium; LA, left atrium; RV, right venricle; LV, left ventricle.

roentgenogram shows (1) no abnormal radiographic findings if left-to-right shunt is small (rare); (2) increased pulmonary vascularity; (3) increased cardiac size; (4) prominent right atrial border (posteroanterior and left anterior oblique projections) because of increased right atrial volume; and (5) fullness of retrosternal space because of right ventricular enlargement.

In patients with complete atrioventricular canal, the following roentgenographic findings are present: (1) marked cardiac enlargement (Fig. 5–43); (2) right atrial enlargement; (3) right ventricular enlargement; (4) increased pulmonary arterial vascularity, and in infants, a superimposed pulmonary edema.

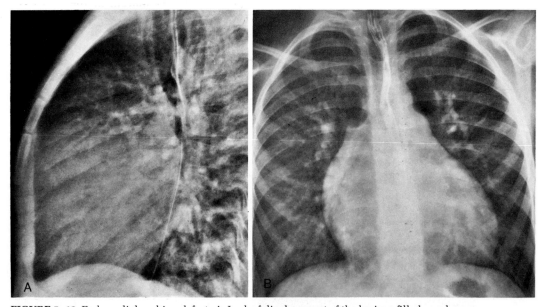

FIGURE 5–42. Endocardial cushion defect. *A*, Lack of displacement of the barium-filled esophagus by the left atrium. Fullness of the retrosternal space produced by the enlarged right ventricle. Hypersegmentation of the sternum. *B*, Increased pulmonary atrial vascularity. Cardiomegaly. Prominent right cardiac border indicates right atrial enlargement. Prominent pulmonary artery segment.

FIGURE 5–43. Complete atrioventricular canal. Markedly increased pulmonary arterial vascularity. Enlarged hilar pulmonary arteries. Haziness of vascular markings. Cardiomegaly. Round, laterally displaced apex. Prominent main pulmonary artery segment.

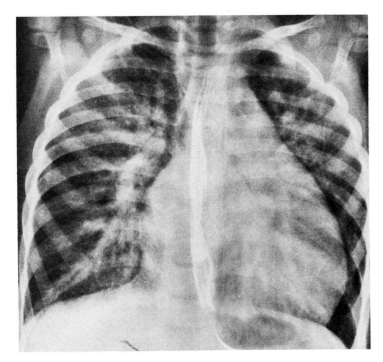

Angiographic Appearance. The angiocardiographic diagnosis of endocardial cushion defect is made by the demonstration of the classic "gooseneck deformity" of the left ventricular outflow tract observed in the anteroposterior projection of a left ventriculogram (Fig. 5–44). This deformity results from the displaced attachment of the septal leaflet of the mitral valve to the lower margin of the

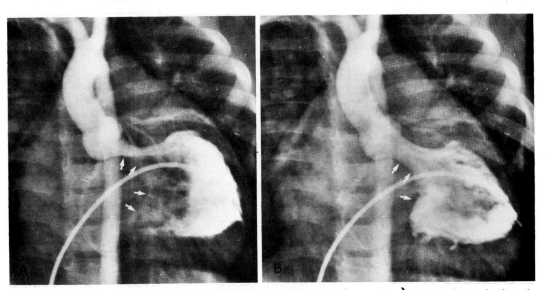

FIGURE 5–44. Endocardial cushion defect. Left ventriculogram in anteroposterior projection. *A*, Diastole. Classic "gooseneck" deformity (arrows) of left ventricular outflow tract. *B*, Systole. "Gooseneck" deformity (arrows) less apparent. Mitral reflux present.

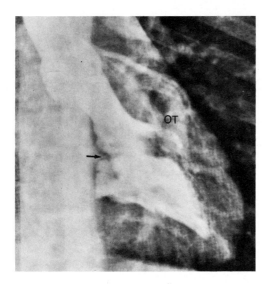

FIGURE 5–45. Endocardial cushion defect. Left ventriculogram. Anteroposterior projection. Cleft (arrow) in mitral valve. Left-to-right shunt at ventricular level. Opacification of right ventricular outflow tract (OT).

endocardial cushion defect. Clefts or serrations in the mitral valve leaflets are also well seen in this projection (Fig. 5–45).

A more complete evaluation of the specific anomalies present in the atrial septum, ventricular septum, and atrioventricular valves can be obtained by a left ventriculogram in the hepatoclavicular projection. In this projection, defects in the posterior ventricular septum are demonstrated; the atrial septum observed in profile and the atrioventricular valves can be separated from one another.

Angiographic findings vary with the type of endocardial cushion defect present.

Partial Atrioventricular Canal

In this form of atrioventricular canal, the ventricular septum is intact and two separate atrioventricular valves are present. Therefore, following left ventriculography, the right ventricle does not opacify immediately. In this view, the cleft in the mitral or tricuspid valves, or both, is clearly seen. Contrast medium refluxes into the left atrium, the amount depending upon the degree of mitral insufficiency. Following opacification of the left atrium, contrast material opacifies the right atrium and subsequently the right ventricle and pulmonary artery. This left-to-right shunt occurs through the ostium primum defect, but the details of the defect may not be clearly demonstrated.

Complete Atrioventricular Canal

A hepatoclavicular projection of a left ventriculogram will demonstrate the presence of a posterior ventricular septal defect, with contrast material immediately opacifying the right ventricle. In this projection, the presence of a common atrioventricular valve is evident as a large round radiolucency overlying both ventricles (Fig. 5–46). In the transitional form of atrioventricular canal, narrow jets of contrast medium can be demonstrated as they pass across the small spaces between the valve leaflets, the superior rim of the ventricular septum, and the short chordae (Fig. 5–47). Clefts in the mitral and tricuspid components of these leaflets can also be easily demonstrated. The amount of reflux from the left

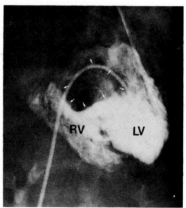

FIGURE 5–46. Complete atrioventricular canal. Left ventriculogram in long-axial oblique projection. Common atrioventricular valve (white arrows). Shunt through ventricular septal defect. LV, left ventricle; RV, right ventricle.

ventricle through the common valve into the left atrium is variable. Commonly the contrast material is seen to pass directly from the left ventricle into the right atrium. There is, in addition, passage of contrast material from the left to the right atrium through the atrial portion of the canal defect. The size of the ostium primum atrial septal defect can be best demonstrated in the hepatoclavicular projection with injection of contrast medium in the right upper pulmonary vein.

Management. Many patients with a partial or transitional form of atrioventricular canal have few symptoms during early childhood. For these patients, operation is performed at preschool age; the ostium primum defect is patched, and usually a mitral valvuloplasty, involving suturing of the cleft, is performed.

Patients with complete atrioventricular canal generally require an operation in infancy. In patients who have a significant amount of mitral insufficiency, a corrective procedure is performed, in which the common valve leaflets are divided, and a patch sewn to close the defect involving the ventricular and atrial septa.

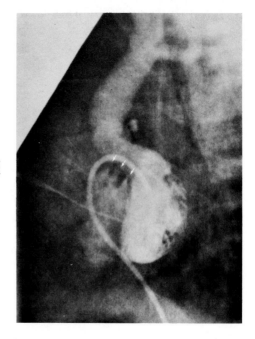

FIGURE 5–47. Transitional type of atrioventricular canal. Left ventriculogram in lateral projection. Multiple small jets through ventricular septal defects (small arrows).

The mitral and tricuspid portions of the common leaflets are then sewn to the patch. This is a detailed operation that is difficult to perform in small infants, and the mortality rate in infants is at least 20 per cent. Therefore, at some centers, patients with complete atrioventricular canal with a large shunt at the ventricular level and minimal mitral insufficiency undergo pulmonary artery banding. Subsequently, around 18 months of age, the band is removed and the malformation corrected.

Other Conditions Without Left Atrial Enlargement

Partial Anomalous Pulmonary Venous Connection. In 10 per cent of patients with atrial septal defect, partial anomalous pulmonary venous connection may coexist. It usually is of the type in which the right upper lobe pulmonary vein connects to the low superior vena cava or to the right atrium near a sinus venosus atrial septal defect. It is difficult to diagnose radiographically or angiographically because the pulmonary veins usually follow a fairly normal course. Occasionally, when they follow a markedly abnormal course, they can be recognized radiographically (Fig. 5–48).

Rarely, PAPVC occurs with an intact atrial septum. The clinical and radiographic findings are identical to those of atrial septal defect.

Selected Bibliography

Barcly, R. S., Reid, J. M., Colman, E. N., Stevenson, J. G., Walsh, T. M., and McSwain, N.: Communication between the left ventricle and right atrium. Thorax, 22:473–477, 1967.

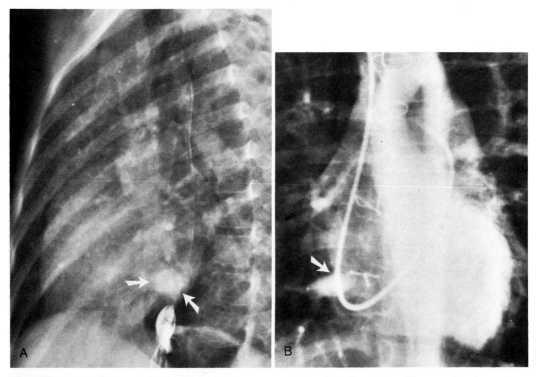

FIGURE 5–48. Partial anomalous pulmonary venous connection. A, Left anterior oblique projection. Abnormal vascular density (arrows) joining posterior cardiac margin. B, Pulmonary arteriogram. Late phase. One pulmonary vein (arrow) from right lower lobe connects to right atrium.

Blieden, L. C., Randall, P. A., Castaneda, A. R., Lucas, R. V., Jr., and Edwards, J. E.: The "goose neck" of the endocardial cushion defect: Anatomic basis. Chest, 65:13–17, 1974.

Cantor, S., Sanderson, R., and Cohn, K.: Left ventricular-right atrial shunt due to bacterial endocarditis. Chest, 60:552–554, 1971.

Dunseth, W., and Ferguson, T.: Acquired cardiac septal defect due to thoracic trauma. Trauma, 5:142–149, 1965.

Rowbin, R., and Schwartz, D.: Endocardial cushion defects: Embryology, anatomy, and angiography. AJR, 136:157–162, 1981.

Shanes, J. G., Levitsky, S., Seyal, M. S., Welch, W., Kondos, G., Silverman, N., Rich, S., and Pietras, R. J.: Diagnosis of left ventricular to right atrial shunt utilizing contrast echocardiography. Am. J. Cardiol., 52:650, 1983.

Silverman, N. A., Sethi, G. K., and Scott, S. M.: Acquired left ventricular-right atrial fistula following aortic valve replacement. Ann. Thorac. Surg., 30:82–486, 1980.

Smallhorn, J. F., Tommasini, G., Anderson, R. H., and Macartney, F. J.: Assessment of atrioventricular septal defects by two dimensional echocardiography. Br. Heart J., 47:109–121, 1982.

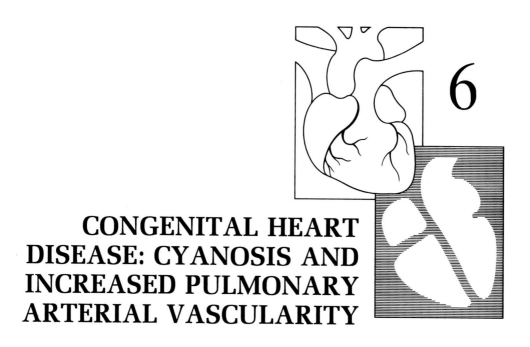

6

CONGENITAL HEART DISEASE: CYANOSIS AND INCREASED PULMONARY ARTERIAL VASCULARITY

The combination of cyanosis and increased pulmonary blood flow is associated with "admixture" lesions, conditions with bidirectional shunting, which in most instances causes uniform mixing of the systemic and pulmonary venous returns. Clinically these patients present with cyanosis and congestive cardiac failure. Delayed growth and recurrent pneumonia are common.

The three most frequently occurring admixture lesions are transposition of great vessels, truncus arteriosus, and total anomalous pulmonary venous connection. *Key*

The radiologist should evaluate the pulmonary artery in the roentgenogram of a patient with an admixture lesion. If it is not present along the upper left cardiac border, a transposition of the great vessels should be considered, since the pulmonary artery is located medially in transposition and not along the left cardiac border. In the other admixture lesions, the main pulmonary artery segment is present and frequently enlarged.

If the pulmonary artery segment is present, the size of the left atrium should be evaluated. If left atrial enlargement is present, it means that the shunt occurs at the ventricular or great vessel level, e.g., truncus arteriosus. If left atrial enlargement is not present, the shunt occurs at the atrial or venous level, e.g., total anomalous pulmonary venous connection.

TRANSPOSITION OF GREAT VESSELS

The term transposition of great vessels indicates that the great vessels originate from the inappropriate ventricle. Thus the aorta originates from the right ventricle and the pulmonary artery from the left ventricle. Generally the aorta lies anterior to the pulmonary artery. *Key*

There are two basic anatomic types of transposition of the great vessels.

egg on side

Rashkind
Blalock-Hanlon
Mustard

Complete Transposition of the Great Vessels

This form of transposition of the great vessels accounts for 10 per cent of the cases of congenital heart disease and is the most common anomaly causing syanosis in neonates.

Anatomic Features. In complete transposition of the great vessels, the aorta arises from the right ventricle and receives systemic venous blood, while the pulmonary artery arises from the left ventricle and receives pulmonary venous blood. As a result, two nearly independent circulations are established; one of blood returning from the body passing through the right side of the heart and being delivered to the body; the other of blood returning to the heart from the lungs and again returning to the lungs through the left side of the heart. This circulatory pattern causes marked hypoxemia and is incompatible with survival, unless there are associated anomalies that permit mixing of the two circulations.

Cases of complete transposition of the great vessels have been classified according to the types of associated malformations that might permit mixing.

1. Intact ventricular septum. Mixing occurs through patent ductus arteriosus and patent foramen ovale.

2. Ventricular septal defect.
   a. Without pulmonary stenosis.
   b. With pulmonary stenosis.

Hemodynamics. The hemodynamics, clinical course, and features vary according to these coexistent conditions.

In patients with an intact atrial septum (Fig. 6–1), the patent ductus carries aortic blood (desaturated blood) into the pulmonary artery, while the patent

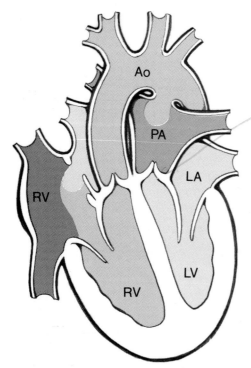

mitral/pulmonic continuity

FIGURE 6–1. The central circulation with complete transposition of the great arteries. Intact ventricular septum. Shunts occur at atrial and ductal levels. Ao, Aorta; LA, left atrium; LV, left ventricle; PA, pulmonary artery; RA, right atrium, RV, right ventricle.

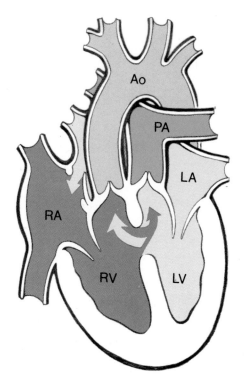

FIGURE 6–2. The central circulation with complete transposition of the great arteries and ventricular septal defect. Bidirectional shunt at ventricular level. Abbreviations as in Figure 6–1.

foramen ovale allows fully saturated blood to flow from the left atrium to the right atrium. The ductus arteriosus usually closes during the first 48 hours of life, leaving the patient with only a patent foramen ovale through which a bidirectional shunt can occur, but which is usually very ineffective. Symptoms of severe hypoxia thus occur within the first two to three days of life, and death ensues shortly unless some type of communication is created to allow intracardiac mixing to occur.

In patients with a coexistent ventricular septal defect, a bidirectional shunt can occur (Fig. 6–2), and this provides better mixing than a patent foramen ovale. Patients with a coexistent ventricular septal defect are usually less cyanotic, but those without pulmonary stenosis tend to develop congestive cardiac failure in a fashion similar to isolated ventricular septal defect. Patients in whom pulmonary stenosis coexists with the ventricular septal defect have the longest survival without treatment, since the pulmonary stenosis limits the volume of pulmonary blood flow and thus prevents congestive cardiac failure. It also favors the shunt of oxygenated blood from the left ventricle to the aorta.

Clinical Features. Most patients, regardless of the type of associated anomalies, develop cyanosis in the neonatal period. The cyanosis may be severe. There may be either no murmur or a soft murmur. In patients with a ventricular septal defect or pulmonary stenosis, or both, the murmur may be louder and more typical of that condition. The second heart sound is loud and single.

In newborns the electrocardiogram is normal, but with age a pattern of right axis deviation and right ventricular hypertrophy develops.

Echocardiographic Features. In M-mode echocardiography the anterior blood vessel (aorta) lies anteriorly to the right in comparison to normal, in which the anterior blood vessel (pulmonary artery) lies anteriorly to the left. The posterior (pulmonary) semilunar valve closes after the anterior (aortic) semilunar valve, opposite the normal pattern. In M-mode, the presence of a ventricular septal

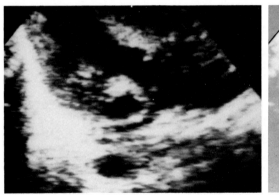
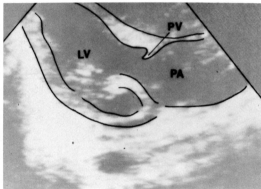

FIGURE 6–3. Complete transposition of the great arteries. Cross-sectional echocardiogram. Long axis projection. Left ventricle connects with pulmonary artery. LV, left ventricle; PV, pulmonary valve; PA, pulmonary artery.

defect may be noted by drop-out of septal echoes, and subpulmonary stenosis by left ventricular outflow tract narrowing and flutter of the pulmonary valve.

Cross-sectional echocardiography allows much better definition of the anomaly, since it is possible to demonstrate the aorta arising from the anterior (right) ventricle, and the pulmonary artery from the posterior (left) ventricle (Figs. 6–3 and 6–4). The echo is also useful in demonstrating the presence of a large ventricular septal defect, the status of the atrial septum, and, with greater difficulty, obstructive lesions in the left ventricular outflow area.

Chest X-ray Features. The chest x-ray is usually typical for complete transposition of the great vessels (Fig. 6–5).

1. The pulmonary vasculature shows a pattern of increased pulmonary arterial markings.

2. The cardiac size is increased.

3. The cardiac contour has been described as an "egg-on-its-side" or "apple-on-a-string." The superior mediastinum is narrow, perhaps because the great vessels lie in front of one another, rather than side by side. The thymus is small. The cardiac contour is oval and lies obliquely (Fig. 6–5).

4. The pulmonary artery segment is absent, since the pulmonary artery lies posteriorly and in the mid-line. It does not form a portion of the cardiac border.

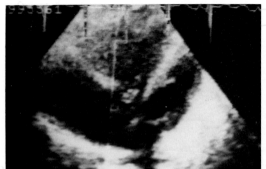
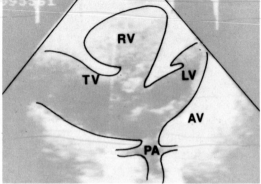

FIGURE 6–4. Complete transposition of the great arteries. Cross-sectional echocardiogram. Subcostal view. Left ventricle gives rise to pulmonary artery. RV, right ventricle; TV, tricuspid valve; LV, left ventricle; AV, aortic valve; PA, pulmonary artery.

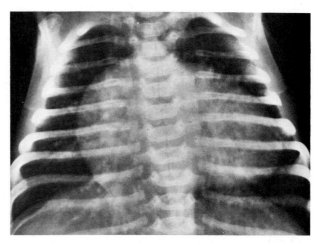

FIGURE 6–5. Complete transposition of the great arteries. Increased pulmonary arterial vascularity. Cardiomegaly, with "egg-on-its-side" configuration. Prominent right cardiac border. Flat pulmonary artery segment.

5. If the pulmonary vascular resistance does not fall significantly after birth, the pulmonary vascularity may appear decreased (Fig. 6–6A). This changes as the pulmonary vascular resistance falls (Fig. 6–6B).

Angiographic Appearance. The diagnosis of complete transposition of the great vessels is best established by right ventriculography. This study demonstrates the origin of the aorta anteriorly from the right ventricle (Fig. 6–7). In the left ventriculogram, the pulmonary artery originates posteriorly from the left ventricle (Fig. 6–8). In these angiograms coexistent conditions can be diagnosed (Fig. 6–8). Subpulmonary or valvular pulmonary stenosis is best demonstrated on a long-axial oblique projection of a left ventriculogram. Ventricular septal defect is demonstrated on a right ventriculogram in a long-axial oblique projection.

Management. Most neonatal patients with complete transposition of the great vessels require emergency treatment. Prostaglandin E_1 is administered intravenously in an effort to maintain ductal patency and improve oxygenation so that the neonates can undergo cardiac catheterization. During catheterization a balloon atrial septostomy (Rashkind procedure) is performed to allow better mixing at the atrial level. The prostaglandins are then discontinued. The state of oxygenation

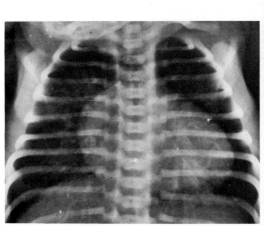
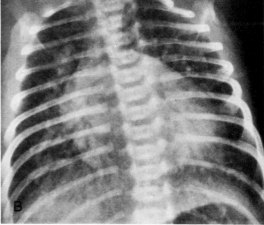

FIGURE 6–6. Complete transposition of the great arteries. A, Slightly increased pulmonary arterial vascularity. Cardiomegaly. Narrow superior mediastinum. B, Increased pulmonary arterial vascularity. Cardiomegaly. Concave pulmonary arterial segment. Narrow superior mediastinum.

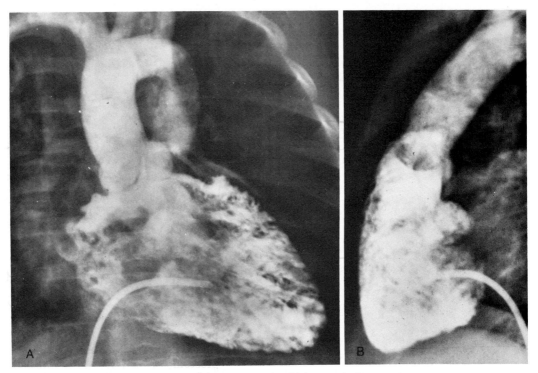

FIGURE 6–7. Complete transposition of the great arteries. Right ventriculogram. *A,* Anteroposterior, and *B,* lateral projections. Aorta arises from the right ventricle.

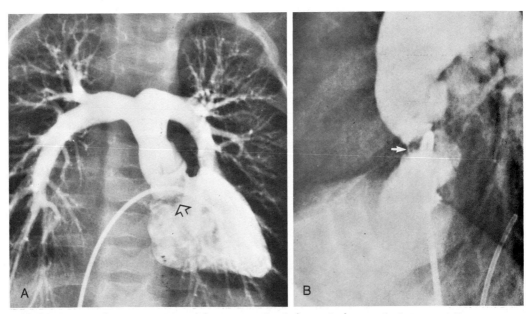

FIGURE 6–8. Complete transposition of the great arteries. Left ventriculogram. *A,* Anteroposterior projection. Pulmonary artery arises from left ventricle. Radiolucent filling defect (arrow) in the outflow tract of the left ventricle represents an area of subpulmonic obstruction. *B,* Lateral projection. Pulmonary artery arises from the left ventricle. Observe severe subpulmonic obstruction (arrow).

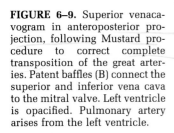

FIGURE 6–9. Superior venacavogram in anteroposterior projection, following Mustard procedure to correct complete transposition of the great arteries. Patent baffles (B) connect the superior and inferior vena cava to the mitral valve. Left ventricle is opacified. Pulmonary artery arises from the left ventricle.

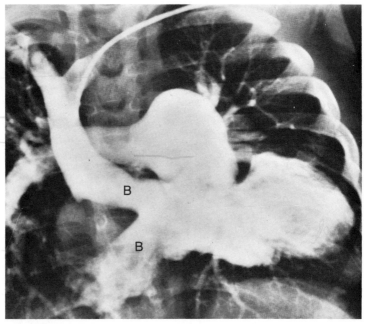

of most infants is improved significantly by the atrial septostomy. An atrial septal defect can also be created by using an operative technique (Blalock-Hanlon procedure).

Later in the first year, a corrective procedure is carried out. An atrial baffle is created, which diverts the systemic venous blood into the left ventricle and the pulmonary venous return into the right ventricle; in this way the circulatory pattern is corrected (Fig. 6–9). Three different operative procedures (Mustard, Senning, or Schumaker procedures) are available. In patients with complete transposition with a ventricular septal defect alone, or with pulmonary stenosis, a conduit type procedure is used for correction.

There has been a recent development in anatomic correction of complete transposition of the great vessels involving division of the aorta and pulmonary arteries above the semilunar valves, attaching them to the opposite great vessel root, and moving the coronary arteries. This procedure must be performed in the neonatal period.

Selected Bibliography

Daskalopoulos, D., Edwards, W. D., Driscoll, D. J., Seward, J. B., Tajik, A. J., and Kagler, D. J.: Correlation of two-dimensional echocardiographic and autopsy findings in complete transposition of the great arteries. J. Am. Coll. Cardiol., *2*(6):1151–1157, 1983.
de la Cruz, M. V., Arteaga, M., Espino-Vela, J., Quero-Jimenez, M., Anderson, R. H., and Diaz, G. F.: Complete transposition of the great arteries: Types and morphogenesis of ventriculararterial discordance. Am. Heart J., *102*:271–281, 1981.
Goor, D. A., and Edwards, J. E.: The spectrum of transposition of the great arteries, with specific reference to developmental anatomy of the conus. Circulation, *48*:406–415, 1973.
Rizk, G., Moller, J. H., and Amplatz, K.: The angiographic appearance of the heart following the Mustard procedure. Radiology, *106*:269–273, 1973.

Congenitally Corrected Transposition of the Great Vessels

This is an uncommon form of transposition of the great vessels, which does not in itself cause cyanosis. The name indicates that the circulatory pattern is

Valves / reversed

correct. That is, the systemic venous blood is delivered to the lungs, pulmonary venous blood is delivered to the body as in normal, and the great vessels are transposed—i.e., the aorta arises from the right ventricle, and the pulmonary artery from the left ventricle. Although the name suggests that the major anomaly lies with the great vessels, the major component is actually inversion of the ventricles. Inversion is a term that indicates a change in lateral relationships, which, when applied to the ventricles, indicates that the anatomic right ventricle lies on the left and the anatomic left ventricle lies on the right.

visceral

atria → situs
Valves → vents

Thus, blood flows from the vena cava into a normally positioned right atrium, and then across a mitral valve into an anatomic left ventricle (Fig. 6–10). The pulmonary artery arises from this ventricle and lies posteriorly to the right of the aorta. The pulmonary venous blood enters the normally positioned left atrium and then crosses a tricuspid valve to enter an anatomic right ventricle. The aorta arises from the infundibulum of this ventricle and lies anteriorly to the left of the pulmonary artery.

bulboventric. loop
rotates wrong
ways!

This condition results from abnormal rotation of the bulboventricular loop during fetal life. Normally, the primitive bulboventricular loop rotates toward the right, so that the right ventricle lies to the right of the left ventricle (Chapter 1). In congenitally corrected transposition of the great vessels, the bulboventricular loop rotates toward the left. This developmental anomaly displaces the right ventricle toward the left, and the left ventricle toward the right.

In most patients with congenitally corrected transposition of the great vessels, other cardiac anomalies coexist. The most common are:

1. Insufficiency of the left atrioventricular (anatomic tricuspid) valve, leading to features of mitral insufficiency.

2. Ventricular septal defect, usually large, with its accompanying features.

3. Pulmonary stenosis, usually coexisting with ventricular septal defect and presenting a clinical picture like that of tetralogy of Fallot.

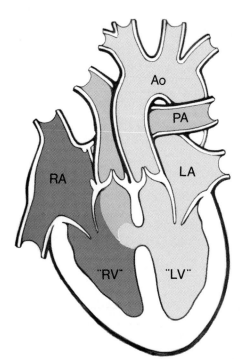

FIGURE 6–10. The central circulation in the presence of congenitally corrected transposition of the great vessels with ventricular septal defect. Left-to-right shunt. Ao, aorta; LA, left atrium; "LV," anatomic left ventricle; PA, pulmonary artery; RA, right atrium; "RV," anatomic right ventricle.

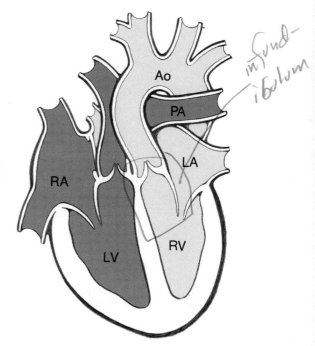

FIGURE 6–11. Central circulation in congenitally corrected transposition of the great vessels. Intact ventricular septum. Abbreviation as in Figure 6–10.

Hemodynamics. The hemodynamic abnormality is that of the associated cardiac condition, anomalies, and is identical to those occurring in patients with normally related great vessels and ventricles (Fig. 6–11).

Clinical Features. The basic clinical features are those of the associated anomaly. There are two features suggesting the underlying condition of corrected transposition of the great vessels: (1) the second heart sound in the pulmonary area is extremely loud and represents closure of the anteriorly located aortic valve, and (2) there is a q wave in lead V_1 and no q wave in lead V_6, the opposite of normal. This pattern indicates inversion of the bundles of His.

Echocardiographic Features. It is difficult to make this diagnosis echocardiographically, since in many patients it is impossible to visualize the interventricular septum because of its orientation in relation to the frontal plane. Continuity between an atrioventricular and semilunar valve on the right side and absence of continuity on the left side are highly suggestive. If the continuity exists in both semilunar valves, the sides are identical. The aortic valve is located anteriorly to the left.

Chest X-ray Findings. The chest x-rays are highly suggestive.

1. The pattern of pulmonary vascularity varies according to the underlying cardiac condition. Cardiac size and pulmonary vascularity may be completely normal.

2. The heart is enlarged in patients with major left atrioventricular valve insufficiency or a large left-to-right shunt. Both of these conditions also cause left atrial enlargement (Fig. 6–12).

3. The cardiac contour is distinctive. Since the pulmonary artery arises medially, it does not form a portion of the cardiac border on a posteroanterior projection. Since the aorta originates and ascends along the upper left cardiac border, the left upper mediastinum is slightly convex. In addition, because of the inverted infundibulum, there is a bulge along the left upper cardiac border, giving a box-shaped configuration (Fig. 6–13).

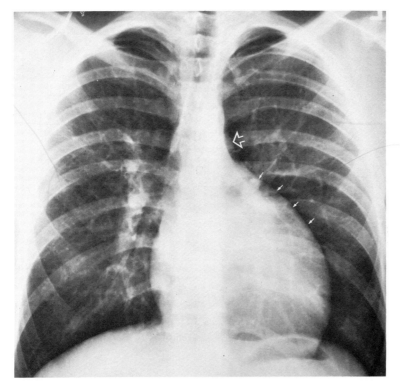

aorta

FIGURE 6–12. Congenitally corrected transposition of the great vessels. Normal pulmonary arterial vascularity. Cardiomegaly. Round prominent left upper cardiac border (small arrows). Extra vascular shadow (open arrow) to the left of the aortic knob represents the ascending aorta. A double density in the area of the left atrium suggests left atrial enlargement.

mitral regurg

2° to ascending aorta

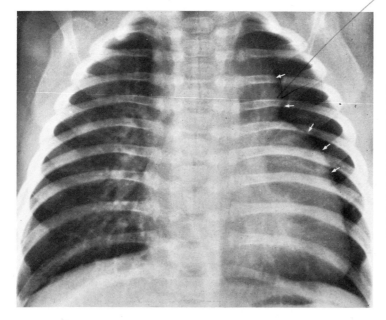

FIGURE 6–13. Congenitally corrected transposition of the great vessels. Increased pulmonary arterial vascularity. Cardiomegaly. Unusual box-shape configuration, produced by a prominence of the left upper cardiac border and prominent upper left mediastinum (arrows). Bulge in left upper cardiac heart border from inverted infundibulum. Prominent upper mediastinum from left-sided ascending aorta.

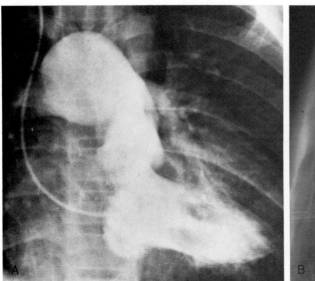
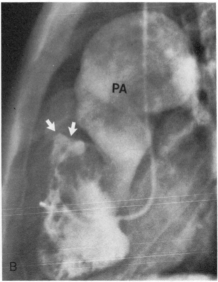

FIGURE 6–14. Anatomic left ventriculogram in congenitally corrected transposition of great vessels. *A,* Anteroposterior projection. Two papillary muscles. Pulmonary artery opacified. Continuity of pulmonary and tricuspid valves. *B,* Lateral projection. Pulmonary artery (PA) is posteriorly positioned. Large anterior shoulder (arrows) of ventricle.

4. Because of the medial displacement of the pulmonary trunk, the right pulmonary artery is well seen and has a "waterfall" appearance.

Angiographic Appearance. The diagnosis can be made angiographically by observing the position of the great vessels and the characteristics of the ventricles. The venous ventricle is a smooth-walled, triangle-shaped chamber. Papillary muscles are easily visualized in this chamber. The pulmonary and atrioventricular valves are in continuity. Thus, there is no infundibulum (Fig. 6–14*A*). In the lateral plane this ventricle lies anteriorly and a smooth shoulder is demonstrated anteriorly and superiorly. The pulmonary artery arising from this ventricle is located posteriorly to the origin of the aorta, and the level of the pulmonary valve is lower than normal because the infundibulum is not present (Fig. 6–14*B*).

Injection into the other ventricle demonstrates the presence of a trabeculated chamber that is located along the left side of the cardiac silhouette. The aortic and atrioventricular valves are not in continuity. There is an infundibular or outflow tract from which the aorta arises. The aorta is positioned anteriorly to the left of the origin of the pulmonary artery. The ascending aorta forms the left upper cardiac border, and this produces the characteristic prominence of the left cardiac border observed on the plain films (Fig. 6–15).

The plane of the ventricular septum, in this condition, is perpendicular to the anteroposterior projection and is easily seen between the ventricles.

Management. In itself, congenitally corrected transposition of the great vessels does not require treatment, but the associated malformations usually require operation. Previously, intracardiac operations were largely avoided because of the complex anatomy and the high incidence of development of complete heart block at operation. Valve replacement of an insufficient left atrioventricular valve was the exception. Palliative procedures, such as banding of the pulmonary artery or creation of a shunt, have often been used when patients were symptomatic. With the development of technique to identify the conduction system intraoperatively, more efforts are now being made to correct the intracardiac anomalies in patients with congenitally corrected transposition of the great vessels.

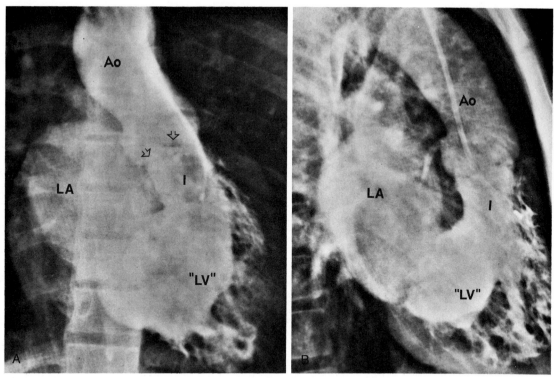

FIGURE 6–15. Anatomic right ventriculogram in congenitally corrected transposition of great vessels. *A,* Anteroposterior projection. Aorta ascends on left side. Infundibulum (I) below aortic valve (open arrows). Atrioventricular valve insufficiency present with opacification of enlarged left atrium. *B,* Lateral projection. Heavy trabeculations. Aorta (Ao) arises anteriorly from infundibulum (I). Massive reflux arises through atrioventricular valve. Dilated left atrium (LA). "LV," anatomic left ventricle.

Selected Bibliography

Anderson, R. C., Lillehei, C. W., and Lester, R. C.: Corrected transposition of the great vessels of the heart. Pediatrics, *20*(4):626–645, 1957.

Hagler, D. J., Tajik, A. J., Seward, J. B., Edwards, W. B., Mair, D. D., and Ritter, D. G.: Atrioventricular and ventriculoarterial discordance (corrected transposition of the great arteries). Mayo Clin. Proc., 56:591–600, 1981.

Lester, R. G., Anderson, R. C., Amplatz, K., and Adams, P.: Roentgenologic diagnosis of congenitally corrected transposition of the great vessels. Am. J. Roentgenol., *83*(6):985–997, 1960.

PERSISTENT TRUNCUS ARTERIOSUS

Persistent truncus arteriosus accounts for 2 per cent of all instances of congenital cardiac anomalies. It results from a failure of formation of the spiral septum within the truncus in the early embryo. As a result, in this anomaly a single arterial vessel (the truncus) leaves the heart and straddles a large ventricular septal defect. The three major arterial circulations, the systemic circulation, the pulmonary circulation, and the coronary circulation arise from the truncus. The right ventricle has no infundibulum. Usually the truncal valve has three semilunar cusps, but less commonly, either two or four. In symptomatic infants, the truncal valve may be stenotic. With age truncal insufficiency develops in one fourth of patients.

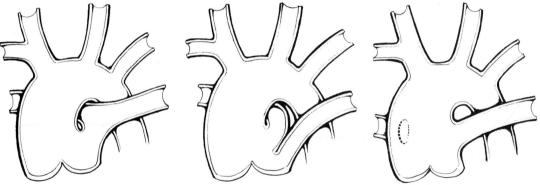

FIGURE 6–16. Types of persistent truncus arteriosus. *Left,* Type I; *Center,* Type II; *Right,* Type III.

Classification. Truncus arteriosus has been classified into four types according to the origin of the pulmonary arteries (Fig. 6–16):

TYPE I   A short main pulmonary artery arises from the left posteriolateral aspect of the truncus and divides into right and left pulmonary arteries.

TYPE II   Each pulmonary artery arises independently from the left posterolateral aspect of the truncus.

TYPE III   Each pulmonary artery arises independently from the lateral aspects of the truncus.

TYPE IV   Pulmonary arteries arise from the descending aorta. All patients with truncus Type IV are probably instances of tetralogy of Fallot with pulmonary atresia. The blood vessels from the descending aorta represent systemic collateral arteries rather than pulmonary arteries.

Since most patients show a form intermediate between I and II, this classification system has been largely abandoned.

Hemodynamics. Truncus arteriosus is an admixture lesion. Both right-to-left and left-to-right shunts occur at the level of the truncus, and the blood becomes fairly uniformly mixed (Fig. 6–17). As in other admixture lesions, the degree of cyanosis is inversely related to the volume of pulmonary blood flow. In truncus the volume of pulmonary blood flow is inversely related to the level of pulmonary vascular resistance. At birth, the level of pulmonary vascular resistance is elevated. Therefore, the volume of pulmonary blood flow is limited, and the neonate with truncus arteriosus shows moderate cyanosis. During infancy, the pulmonary vascular resistance falls normally, and therefore the volume of pulmonary blood flow shows a reciprocal increase. As a result the degree of cyanosis lessens. Because of the excessive volume of pulmonary blood flow, the left ventricle dilates and congestive heart failure develops. Since the ventricular septal defect is large, the systolic pressures are identical in the truncus arteriosus and both ventricles. Pressures in the aorta and pulmonary arteries are also identical, in most cases, since the origin of the pulmonary arteries from the truncus is usually not stenotic. Pulmonary vascular disease develops if the patient is not operated on. As pulmonary vascular disease develops, the volume of pulmonary blood flow decreases and cyanosis increases.

Clinical Features. Patients with persistent truncus arteriosus present with cyanosis and cardiac failure in infancy. There is a systolic murmur similar to a ventricular septal defect. A systolic ejection click and single second heart sound are characteristic. If truncal insufficiency is present, there is an early diastolic murmur of regurgitation. The pulse pressure is wide, and the peripheral pulses sharp, as in other aortic runoff lesions.

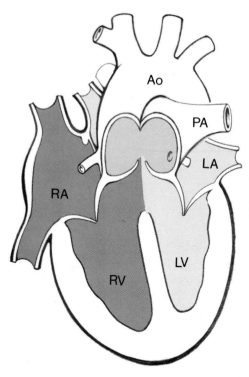

FIGURE 6–17. Central circulation in persistent truncus arteriosus. Bidirectional shunt occurs into truncus. Ao, Aorta; LA, left atrium; LV, left ventricle; PA, pulmonary artery; RA, right atrium; RV, right ventricle.

The electrocardiogram often shows a pattern of biventricular hypertrophy. Right ventricular hypertrophy reflects the elevated right ventricular systolic pressure. Left ventricular hypertrophy reflects the volume overload occurring from either a large volume of pulmonary blood flow or truncal insufficiency.

Echocardiographic Findings. The anterior border of the aortic root is located anteriorly to the plane of the interventricular septum, but continuity between the posterior aortic wall and anterior leaflet of the mitral valve is maintained (Fig. 6–18). There is drop-out of echoes beneath the semilunar valve. The right ventricular anterior wall is thickened. The dimensions of the left atrium and left ventricle increase with the increased pulmonary blood flow. The single great vessel that is visualized is dilated.

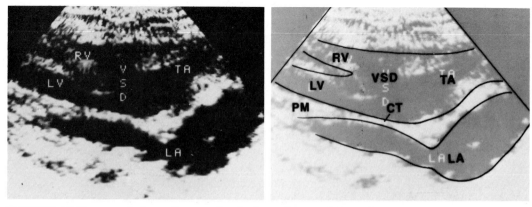

FIGURE 6–18. Truncus arteriosus. Cross-sectional echocardiogram. Subcostal projection. Truncus arteriosus (TA) arises over ventricular septal defect (VSD). Distinct pulmonary artery not visualized. CT, Chordae tendineae; PM, papillary muscle; RV, right ventricle; LV, left ventricle; LA, left atrium.

Selected Bibliography

Becker, A. E., Becker, M. J., and Edwards, J. E.: Pathology of the semilunar valve in persistent truncus arteriosus. J. Thorac. Cardiovasc. Surg., 62(1):16–26, 1971.

Ceballos, R., Soto, B., Kirklin, J. W., and Bargeron, L. M., Jr.: Truncus arteriosus: An anatomical-angiographic study. Br. Heart J., 49:589–599, 1983.

Marin-Garcia, J., and Tonkin, I. L. D.: Two-dimensional echocardiographic evaluations of persistent truncus arteriosus. Am. J. Cardiol., 50:1376–1379, 1982.

TOTAL ANOMALOUS PULMONARY VENOUS CONNECTION

Total anomalous pulmonary venous connection accounts for 2 per cent of congenital cardiac anomalies. It is classified as an admixture lesion because of the combination of cyanosis and increased pulmonary vascularity on the chest x-ray. In common with other admixture lesions, there is both a left-to-right shunt and a right-to-left shunt.

Anatomy. In total anomalous pulmonary venous connection, the incorporation of pulmonary veins into the left atrium does not occur because the common pulmonary vein fails to form during embryonic development. As a result, the confluence of pulmonary veins retains a connection to the primitive systemic venous system. There are four major anatomic forms of total anomalous pulmonary venous connection that can develop.

1. Connection to the superior vena cava (Fig. 6–22)—persistence of communication to the right anterior cardinal system.

2. Connection to the coronary sinus (Fig. 6–23)—persistence of communication to the proximal part of the left anterior cardinal system.

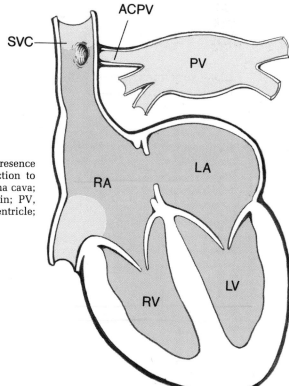

FIGURE 6–22. The central circulation in the presence of total anomalous pulmonary venous connection to the right superior vena cava. SVC, Superior vena cava; ACPV, anaomalous connective pulmonary vein; PV, pulmonary veins; RA, right atrium; RV, right ventricle; LA, left atrium; LV, left ventricle.

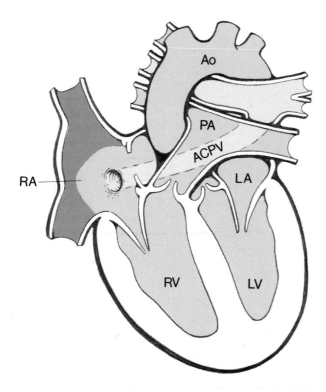

FIGURE 6–23. Central circulation with total anomalous pulmonary venous connection to a coronary sinus. Ao, aorta; LA, left atrium; LV, left ventricle; PA, pulmonary artery; RA, right atrium; RV, right ventricle; ACPV, anomalous connecting pulmonary vein.

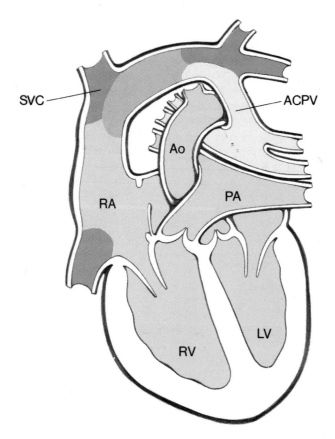

FIGURE 6–24. Central circulation in total anomalous pulmonary venous connection to the left superior vena cava. Ao, aorta; LA, left atrium, LV, left ventricle; PA, pulmonary artery; RA, right atrium; RV, right ventricle; SVC, superior vena cava; ACPV, anomalous connecting pulmonary vein.

3. Connection to the left superior vena cava (Fig. 6–24)—persistence of communication to the distal part of the left anterior cardinal vein.

4. Connection to the portal venous system (Fig. 6–25)—persistence of communication to the umbilical-vitelline system.

An interatrial communication is an integral component. In most forms there is dilatation of the right atrium and right ventricle.

In three fourths of patients the pulmonary venous pathway is unobstructed, but in the other one fourth of patients, particularly those with connection to the portal venous system, either an extrinsic or an intrinsic lesion narrows the pulmonary venous connection.

Hemodynamics. In total anomalous pulmonary venous connection, the entire system and pulmonary venous returns empty into the right atrium where mixing occurs (Figs. 6–22 to 6–25). Blood flows from the right atrium in two directions: into the right ventricle and ultimately into the pulmonary artery, and through the atrial septal defect into the left atrium and ultimately the aorta. The magnitude

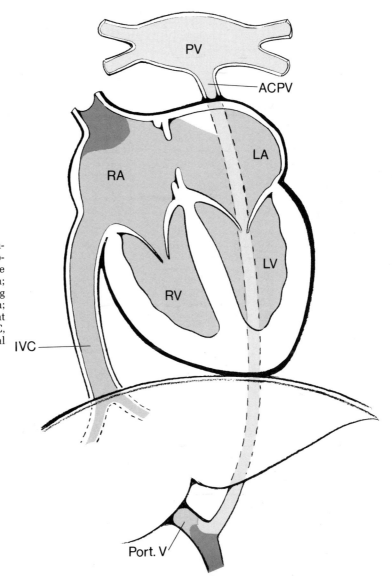

FIGURE 6–25. Central circulation in total anomalous pulmonary venous connection to the portal vein. PV, Pulmonary vein; ACPV, anomalous connecting pulmonary vein; LA, left atrium; LV, left ventricle; RA, right atrium; RV, right ventricle; IVC, inferior vena cava; Port. V, portal vein.

of these flows depends upon the relative ventricular compliances. Since right ventricular compliance is usually considerably less than left ventricular compliance, flow into the right ventricle is greatly increased.

As in other admixture lesions, cyanosis is present, but its severity is inversely related to the volume of pulmonary blood flow.

Clinical Features. There are two clinical and radiographic presentations of total anomalous pulmonary venous connection, depending upon whether or not obstruction occurs in the pathway of pulmonary venous return.

1. Without pulmonary venous obstruction. Cyanosis is present at birth and improves as right ventricular compliance increases secondary to the normal neonatal decrease in pulmonary vascular resistance. Many infants with this condition develop congestive cardiac failure, slow growth, and frequent respiratory infections. The auscultatory findings are similar to those of atrial septal defect. There is a pulmonary systolic ejection murmur; wide, fixed splitting of the second heart sound; and a tricuspid mid-diastolic murmur.

The electrocardiogram resembles atrial septal defect, showing right-axis deviation, right atrial enlargement, and an incomplete right bundle-branch block pattern (rSR′ in lead V_1).

2. With pulmonary venous obstruction. This clinical radiographic picture resembles that of a neonate with parenchymal pulmonary disease. There is intense cyanosis and respiratory distress. There are no cardiac murmurs. The electrocardiogram resembles that of a normal newborn.

Echocardiographic Features. The M-mode echocardiogram of a newborn with total anomalous pulmonary venous connection is normal. On the other hand, infants and children show: (1) dilated right ventricle, (2) paradoxical septal motion, and (3) relatively small left atrium, left ventricle, and aorta (Fig. 6–26). It may be possible to visualize an echo-free cavity immediately behind the left atrium.

With two-dimensional echocardiography in normal neonates, it is usually possible to identify the entry of pulmonary veins into the left atrium. Failure to do so does not constitute a diagnosis of TAPVC but is highly supicious.

Radiographic Features.
1. Without pulmonary venous obstruction. The overall radiographic findings are fairly uniform (Fig. 6–27).
   a. There are increased pulmonary arterial vascular markings.

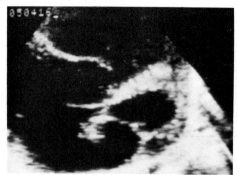
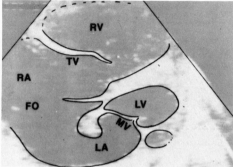

FIGURE 6–26. Cross-sectional echocardiogram. Subcostal four-chamber view. Total anomalous pulmonary venous connection. Dilated right ventricle (RV), and right atrium (RA). Small left atrium (LA) and left ventricle (LV). TV, tricuspid valve; MV, mitral valve; FO, foramen ovale.

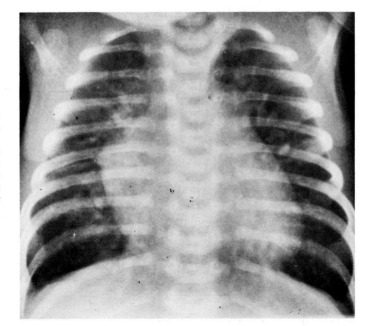

FIGURE 6–27. Total anomalous pulmonary venous connection without pulmonary venous obstruction. Increased pulmonary arterial vascularity. Cardiomegaly. Prominent right atrium. Dilated main pulmonary artery segment. Cardiac apex elevated from right ventricular enlargement.

    b. Cardiomegaly is present, exclusively from right atrial and right ventricular enlargement.
    c. The pulmonary arterial segment is prominent.
    d. The left atrial enlargement is absent, in contrast to most admixture lesions.

There may be cardiac contours that are characteristic of a specific anatomic form of total anomalous pulmonary venous connection.
    a. Connection to left superior vena cava—"snowman heart," "figure-of-eight." The enlarged supracardiac veins, left superior vena cava, innominate vein, and right superior vena cava are dilated and cause a large supracardiac shadow (Fig. 6–28).
    b. Connection to right superior vena cava. The right superior vena cava is dilated and appears enlarged along the upper right cardiac border on thoracic roentgenogram.
    c. Connection to coronary sinus. On a lateral thoracic roentgenogram with barium swallow, the dilated coronary sinus causes a localized indentation of the esophagus at a site lower than the left atrium.
2. With pulmonary venous obstruction (Fig. 6–29).
    a. Increased pulmonary venous markings.
    b. Fine reticular pattern of pulmonary edema throughout both lung fields—resembling neonatal parenchymal pulmonary disease.
    c. Normal cardiac size.
    d. Absent left atrial enlargement.
    e. No dilated pulmonary venous channel, since the volume of pulmonary blood flow is limited by the obstruction.

    Angiographic Appearance. Although anomalous connection of the pulmonary veins can be demonstrated by a right ventriculogram or a pulmonary arteriogram, a more precise anatomic demonstration can be obtained by selective injections in the right or left pulmonary arteries with balloon occlusion. A more precise demonstration can be obtained by selective catheterization and injection of the anomalously connecting veins.

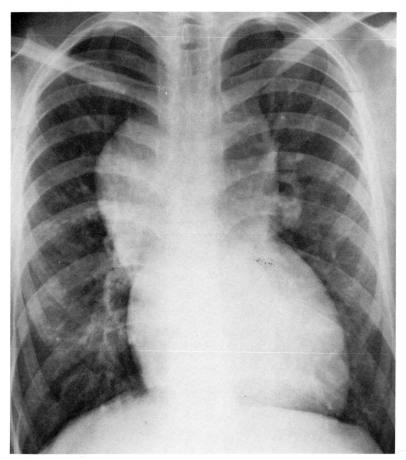

FIGURE 6–28. Total anomalous pulmonary venous connection to left superior vena cava. Increased pulmonary arterial vascularity. Cardiomegaly. Wide upper mediastinum producing the characteristic "snowman" configuration.

Different angiographic pictures are obtained, depending upon the type of anomalous pulmonary venous connection.

1. Connection to left superior vena cava. Following opacification of pulmonary veins, an ascending vein, the innominate vein, the superior vena cava, and the right atrium are successively opacified (Fig. 6–30). Each is markedly dilated. The dilatation of these venous channels causes a widening of the superior mediastinal silhouette, producing the typical radiographic appearance of "snowman" heart.

2. Connection to the right superior vena cava. The venous channel connects to a dilated right superior vena cava (Fig. 6–31).

3. Connection to the coronary sinus. The anomalously connected venous channel drains into the coronary sinus, which is dilated and lies posteriorly in a lateral view. Because of the dilution of contrast material and the presence of overlying opacified structures, such as right and left atrium, this anatomic form may be difficult to diagnose.

4. Connection to infradiaphragmatic site. A long, narrow channel passes inferiorly through the diaphragm and opacifies a portion of the portal system (Fig. 6–32).

In patients with pulmonary venous obstruction the site of obstruction to blood flow is not commonly demonstrated in the infradiaphragmatic types. In the

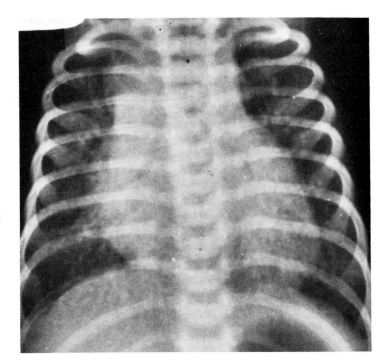

FIGURE 6–29. Total anomalous pulmonary venous connection with pulmonary venous obstruction. Increased pulmonary vascularity with congestive pattern. Cardiomegaly. Enlarged right cardiac border suggests right atrial enlargement.

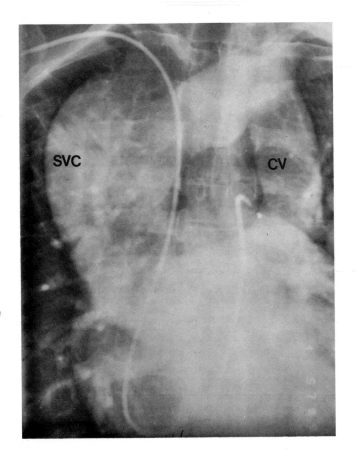

FIGURE 6–30. Total anomalous pulmonary venous connection to left superior vena cava. Late phase of pulmonary arteriogram. Connection of all pulmonary veins to enlarged common pulmonary vein (CV), which connects to innominate vein. Marked dilatation of superior vena cava (SVC).

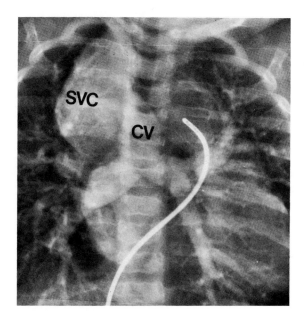

FIGURE 6–31. Total anomalous pulmonary venous connection to right superior vena cava. Late phase of pulmonary arteriogram. Confluence of pulmonary veins drains to markedly dilated superior vena cava (SVC). CV, common pulmonary vein.

supradiaphragmatic types with obstruction, the site may be demonstrated, as when the connecting vein passes between the pulmonary artery and the mainstem bronchus. The narrowing at this site can be observed on a lateral projection.

There are other abnormal angiographic findings reflecting changes in other cardiac structures. Enlargement of the right atrium and right ventricle due to volume overload is present. The left atrium is smaller than normal and right-to-left shunting at the atrial level is present. Because of increased pulmonary blood flow, the pulmonary artery segment is dilated.

Management. Total anomalous pulmonary venous connection is treated by an operation involving three steps: (1) creation of an opening between the confluence of pulmonary veins and the left atrium, (2) closure of the atrial septal

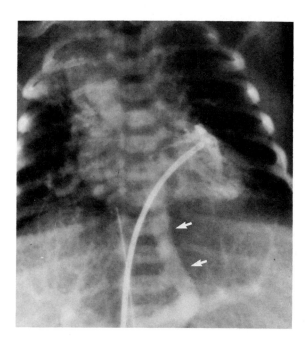

FIGURE 6–32. Asplenia syndrome, common ventricle, and total anomalous pulmonary venous return, below the diaphragm. Late phase of right ventriculogram. Large venous channel (arrows) passes through the diaphragm to connect with the portal vein. Transverse liver.

defect, and (3) ligation of the vein connecting to the systemic venous system. The operation is performed in symptomatic infants or, electively, in asymptomatic patients by one year of age.

Selected Bibliography

Carey, L. S., and Edwards, J. E.: Severe pulmonary venous obstruction in total anomalous pulmonary venous connection to the left innominate vein. Am. J. Roentgenol., *90*(3):593–598, 1963.

Lucas, R. V., Anderson, R. C., Amplatz, K., Adams, P., and Edwards, J. E.: Congenital causes of pulmonary venous obstruction. Pediatr. Clin. North Am., *10*(3):781–836, 1963.

Lucas, R. V., Jr., Adams, P., Jr., Anderson, R. C., Varco, R. L., Edwards, J. E., and Lester, R. G.: Total anomalous pulmonary venous connection to the portal venous system: A cause of pulmonary venous obstruction. Am. J. Roentgenol., *86*(3):561–575, 1961.

Snider, A. R., Silverman, N. H., and Turley, K.: Evaluation of infradiaphragmatic total anomalous pulmonary venous connection with two-dimensional echocardiography. Circulation, *66*(5):1129–1132, 1982.

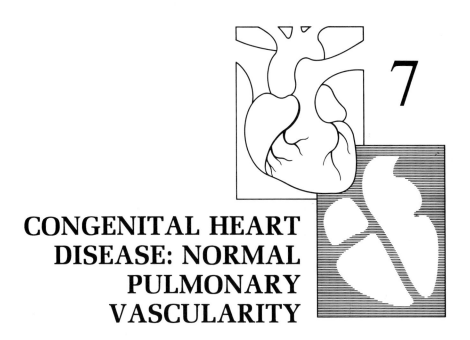

7

CONGENITAL HEART DISEASE: NORMAL PULMONARY VASCULARITY

Among patients with congenital cardiac anomalies, normal pulmonary vascularity is classically associated with lesions causing either outflow obstruction or valvular insufficiency.

Outflow obstruction—aortic stenosis, coarctation of the aorta, interruption of the aortic arch, and pulmonary stenosis—will be discussed in this chapter. Conditions associated with valvular insufficiency also have normal pulmonary vascularity, but are discussed in Chapter 12.

The cardiac size in patients with outflow obstruction may be either normal or enlarged. The former is present in most patients, while the latter is found in either symptomatic infants or older patients with left ventricular failure. Those symptomatic infants with coarctation of the aortic or aortic stenosis may present a pattern of pulmonary venous obstruction, while occasionally an infant with severe pulmonary stenosis may develop a right-to-left shunt through a patent foramen ovale; the pulmonary vascular markings are diminished.

AORTIC STENOSIS

Aortic stenosis accounts for 6 per cent of congenital heart disease in children and may exist as valvular aortic stenosis, subvalvular aortic stenosis, or supravalvular aortic stenosis. The hemodynamic and clinical consequences are similar despite the location of outflow obstruction.

Valvular aortic stenosis (Fig. 7–1) results from: (1) bicuspid aortic valve (most common form), in which two aortic leaflets are present and stenosis results from commissural fusion; and (2) unicommissural valve, in which a single valve leaflet is shaped like a horseshoe. In the latter, stenosis results from the shape of the valve, fusion of the single commissure, and thickening of the cusp.

Subvalvular stenosis results from (1) discrete membranous subaortic stenosis, in which a fibrous ring encircles the immediate subaortic area, and (2) hypertrophic

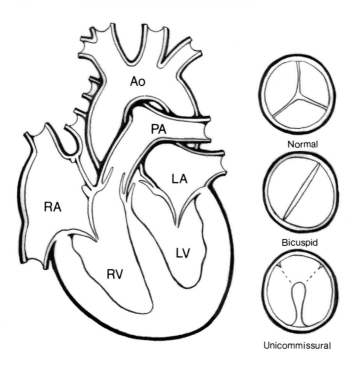

FIGURE 7–1. Central circulation in valvular aortic stenosis. Ao, Aorta; LA, left atrium; LV, left ventricle; PA, pulmonary artery; RA, right atrium; RV, right ventricle.

muscular subaortic stenosis, a myocardial disease causing dynamic subaortic obstruction by contraction of the hypertrophied septum and anterior motion of the septal leaflet of the mitral valve.

Supravalvular aortic stenosis results from an hourglass deformity of the ascending aorta as part of a generalized arteriopathy that may involve other major vessels, particularly the coronary, brachiocephalic, and pulmonary arteries.

Hemodynamics. Regardless of anatomic form, left ventricular outflow obstruction leads to predictable effects (Fig. 7–1). One is turbulence of blood flow through the obstruction. The turbulence produces murmurs and can cause post-stenotic dilatation. Whereas both valvular aortic stenosis and coarctation of the aorta show post-stenotic dilatation, subvalvular and supravalvular do not. In subvalvular aortic stenosis the jet of blood passing through the subaortic stenosis strikes the aortic valve leaflets and its energy is dissipated; in supravalvular aortic stenosis the aorta is intrinsicaly narrowed by the disease process.

The second effect of left ventricular outflow obstruction is an increase in left ventricular systolic pressure, proportional to the degree of stenosis. The left venricle compensates for the obstruction by the development of concentric hypertrophy, not by enlargement. Left ventricular myocardial oxygen requirements are increased because of the left ventricular hypertrophy. If the oxygen requirements are unmet, myocardial ischemia and fibrosis may develop in the left ventricle. Coronary blood flow is normal, except in patients with supravalvular aortic stenosis, in whom the coronary artery may be narrowed.

With considerable left ventricular fibrosis, left ventricular dilatation and ultimately congestive heart failure may develop.

Clinical Features. Most patients are asymptomatic. A few develop congestive heart failure in infancy. Anginal chest pain and syncope occur in children with severe stenosis and myocardial ischemia.

There is an aortic systolic ejection murmur, often associated with a suprasternal notch thrill. A systolic ejection click is present in valvular aortic stenosis because of the post-stenotic dilatation. Patients with a bicuspid aortic valve or with subaortic stenosis may have a murmur of aortic insufficiency.

The electrocardiogram may be normal or may show a pattern of left ventricular hypertrophy. ST segment and T wave changes in the left precordial leads suggest myocardial ischemia; these abnormalities have been associated with angina and sudden death.

Echocardiographic Features. The left ventricle has a thickened wall. In valvular aortic stenosis, there are multiple diastolic echoes from the aortic leaflets and often eccentric closure of the valve in diastole. In cross-sectional recording, movement of the valve leaflets is limited (Fig. 7–2).

In subaortic stenosis a band of echoes may be found beneath the aortic valve. There is asymmetrical opening of the aortic valve cusps, because of the subaortic jet, and partial closure of the aortic valve leaflets early in systole.

In supravalvular aortic stenosis two-dimensional echocardiography can visualize the ascending aorta and brachiocephalic arteries. The hourglass deformity of the ascending aorta can be identified and the narrowing of carotid or subclavian arteries visualized.

Radiographic Features

1. The pulmonary vascularity is normal.

2. Cardiac size is usually normal. In the compensated stage the left ventricular hypertrophy produces a round, slightly up-tilted apex (Fig. 7–3).

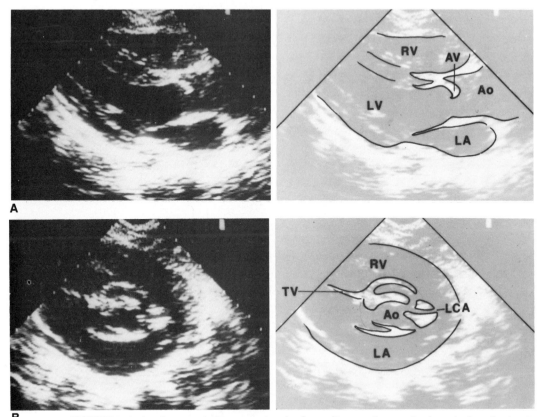

FIGURE 7–2. Aortic stenosis. Cross-sectional echocardiogram. Long-axis view. *A,* Systole. Aortic valve (AV) domes. *B,* Short-axis view. Two leaflets of bicuspid aortic valve observed. Ao, Aorta; LA, left atrium; LV, left ventricle; RV, right ventricle; TV, tricuspid valve; LCA, left coronary artery.

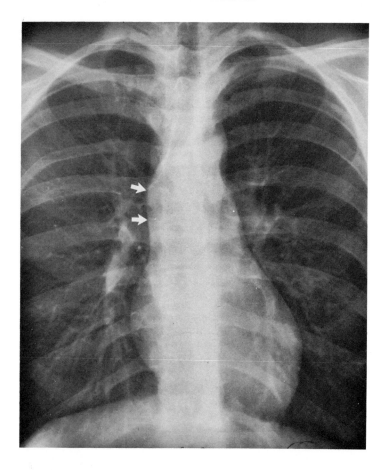

FIGURE 7–3. Aortic valvular stenosis. Normal pulmonary vascularity. Normal cardiac size. Round left cardiac border. Prominent ascending aorta (arrows).

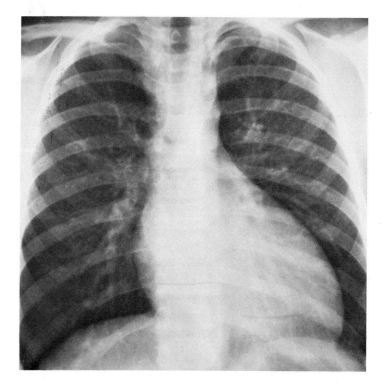

FIGURE 7–4. Aortic valvular stenosis with aortic insufficiency. Normal pulmonary arterial vascularity. Cardiomegaly. Left ventricular configuration, with downward and lateral displacement of cardiac apex.

3. With the development of arotic insufficiency or cardiac decompensation, the cardiac silhouette may have a left ventricular contour with a rounded and elongated appearance of the left cardiac border. The cardiac apex is displaced downward (Fig. 7–4).

4. In valvular aortic stenosis post-stenotic dilatation of the ascending aorta is present, located along the anterior and lateral aortic walls where the jet strikes. The dilatation causes prominence of the upper right cardiac border, which is best observed in posteroanterior and left anterior oblique projection (Fig. 7–5). Post-stenotic dilatation is found in half of the patients with discrete subvalvular stenosis.

5. The size of the aortic knob appears normal, except in supravalvular aortic stenosis where it is small because of aortic hypoplasia.

6. Cardiomegaly and pulmonary edema occur in infants with severe aortic stenosis; congestive cardiac failure results (Fig. 7–6).

7. Cardiomegaly is rarely found in older children.

Angiographic Appearance. Aortography with injection into the root of the aorta is the best method to demonstrate the valvular abnormality. The aortic valve domes, because the fusion of the commissures limits their mobility (Fig. 7–7). During systole the aortic valve leaflets are visualized, in contrast to normal when the valve leaflets are not seen during systole. The sizes of the sinuses of Valsalva are unequal in patients with a bicuspid valve. In these patients there is a large posterior non-coronary sinus and a smaller conjoined anterior sinus above which the coronary arteries arise. Post-stenotic dilatation of the ascending aorta is commonly present (Fig. 7–7). The width of the jet of contrast material across

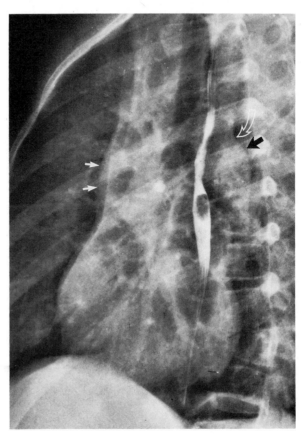

FIGURE 7–5. Aortic valvular stensuis. Prominent ascending aorta (white arrows). Left cardiac border overlaps spine, indicating left ventricular enlargement. Post-stenotic dilatation of descending aorta (large black arrow) beyond coexistent coarctation of the aorta (large curved open arrow).

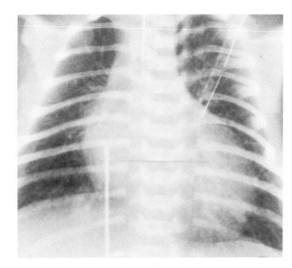

FIGURE 7–6. Aortic valvular stenosis with cardiac failure. Congestive pattern in both lungs. Cardiomegaly with a left ventricular configuration.

the aortic valve can be measured but is usually of little value in assessing the degree of aortic obstruction. A long-axial oblique is the best projection for the study of this condition, since it adequately demonstrates the plane of the aortic valve and, if aortic insufficiency is associated, allows the study of the subaortic area.

A subaortic membrane can be well demonstrated in the AP projection using caudal beam angulation, or in the left anterior oblique projection with cranial beam angulation. A subaortic membrane is usually located a few millimeters below the aortic valve and is evident as a thin radiolucent line (Fig. 7–8). Dynamic subaortic obstruction can also be demonstrated in this projection and shows apposition of the anterior mitral valve leaflet with the ventricular septum during systole. This is better demonstrated in the left anterior oblique projection.

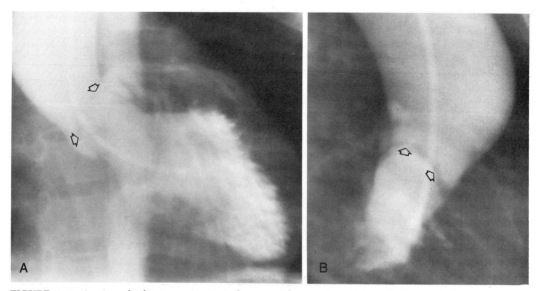

FIGURE 7–7. Aortic valvular stenosis. *A,* Left ventriculogram in anteroposterior projection. Enlarged left ventricle. Doming of aortic valve leaflets (arrows). *B,* Aortogram. Anteroposterior projection. Doming of aortic valve (open arrows). Marked post-stenotic dilatation of ascending aorta.

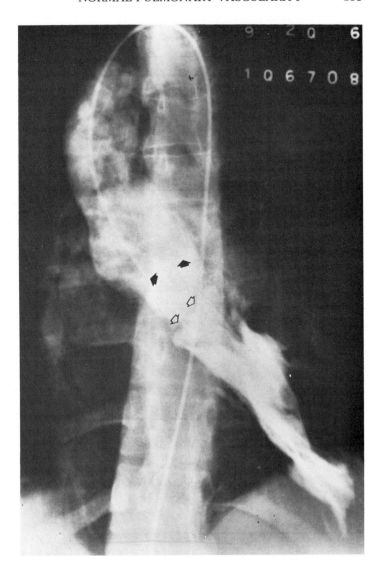

FIGURE 7–8. Subaortic stenosis. Left ventriculogram in a shallow left anterior oblique projection. Thin radiolucent line (open arrows) across left ventricular outflow tract below aortic valve (black arrows).

Supravalvular aortic stenosis is well demonstrated by injections into the root of the aorta. An hourglass deformity is usually located in the ascending aorta and may extend around the aortic arch. The coronary arteries may be narrowed and the brachiocephalic arteries, which may also be narrowed in this condition, can also be assessed by aortography (Fig. 7–9).

Management. Most children with valvular aortic stenosis undergo aortic valvotomy as teenagers, even though they are asymptomatic. Congestive cardiac failure or significant symptoms are definite indications for operation.

Valvotomy can be performed successfully in children and can yield satisfactory results, since the leaflets are pliable and not calcified. Usually by the age of 20 years the valve leaflets are rigid enough to require valve replacement.

Discrete subaortic stenosis is treated by resection of the subaortic membrane using an approach through the ascending aorta and the aortic valve.

Supravalvular stenosis is operated upon by making a longitudinal incision across the stenotic area and widening the area with a patch.

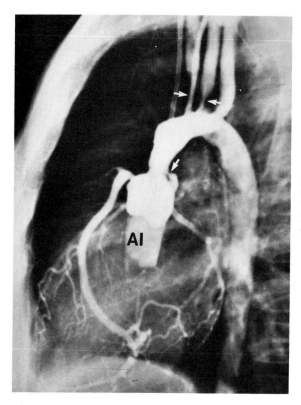

FIGURE 7–9. Supravalvular aortic stenosis. Aortogram in lateral projection. Dilated sinuses of Valsalva. Narrowed ascending aorta. Narrowed origin (arrows) of left coronary artery and of brachiocephalic arteries. Aortic insufficiency (AI).

Selected Bibliography

Valvular Aortic Stenosis

Brandenburg, R. O., Jr., Tajik, A., J., Edwards, E. D., Reeder, G. S., Shub, C., and Seward, J. B.: Accuracy of two-dimensional echocardiographic diagnosis of congenitally bicuspid aortic valve: Echocardiographic-anatomic correlation in 115 patients. Am. J. Cardiol., 51(9):1469–1473, 1983.

Edwards, J. E.: Pathology of left ventricular outflow tract obstruction. Circulation, 31:586–599, 1965.

Finegan, R. E., Gianelly, R. E., and Harrison, D. C.: Aortic stenosis in the elderly: Relevance of age to diagnosis and treatment. N. Engl. J. Med., 1261–1262, 1969.

Hufnagel, C. A., and Conrad, P. W.: Calcific aortic stenosis. N. Engl. J. Med., 266(2);72–76, 1962.

Jarchow, B. H., and Kincaid, O. W.: Poststenotic dilatation of the ascending aorta: Its occurrence and significance as a roentgenologic sign of aortic stenosis. Proc. Staff Meet. Mayo Clin., 36(2):23–33, 1961.

Lababidi, Z., Wu, J.-R., and Walls, J. T.: Percutaneous balloon aortic valvuloplasty: Results in 23 patients. Am. J. Cardiol., 53:194–197, 1984.

Moller, J. H., Nakib, A., Eliot, R. S., and Edwards, J. E.: Symptomatic congenital aortic stenosis in the first year of life. J. Pediatr., 69(5):728–734, 1966.

Supravalvular Aortic Stenosis

Beuren, A. J., Schulze, D., Eberle, P., Harmjanz, D., and Apitz, J.: The syndrome of supravalvular aortic stenosis, peripheral pulmonary stenosis, mental retardation and similar facial appearance. Am. J. Cardiol., 13:471–483, 1964.

Flaker, G., Teske, D., Kilman, J., Hosier, D., and Wooley, C.: Supravalvular aortic stenosis: A 20-year clinical perspective and experience with patch aortoplasty. Am. J. Cardiol., 51:256–260, 1983.

Subaortic Stenosis

Maron, B. J., Tajik, A. J., Ruttenberg, H. D., Graham, T. P., Atwood, G. F., Victorica, B. E., Lie, J. T., and Roberts, W. C.: Hypertrophic cardiomyopathy in infants: Clinical features and natural history. Circulation, 65(1):7–17, 1982.

Olsen, E. G. J.: The pathology of idiopathic hypertrophic subaortic stenosis (hypertrophic cardiomy-opathy). A critical review. Am. Heart J., *100*(4):553–562, 1980.

Shem-Tov, A., Schneeweiss, A., Motro, M., and Neufeld, H. N.: Clinical presentation and natural history of mild discrete subaortic stenosis: Follow-up of 1–17 years. Circulation, *66*(3):509–512, 1982.

Wilcox, W. D., Seward, J. B., Hagler, D. J., Mair, D. D., and Tajik, A. J.: Discete subaortic stenosis: Two-dimensional echocardiographic features with angiographic and surgical correlation. Mayo Clin. Proc., *55*:425–433, 1980.

COARCTATION OF THE AORTA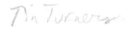

In coarctation of the aorta a localized obstruction exists at the junction of the aortic arch and the descending aorta. A fibrous ridge protrudes into the aorta, narrowing its orifice. A sharp indentation is present in the lateral aortic wall at the coarctation site. Virtually all coarctations occur opposite the ductus. In half of the patients a bicuspid aortic valve coexists.

Coarctation of the aorta may be divided into two anatomic and hemodynamic types. (1) Aortic isthmus narrowing. In addition to the localized constriction, the aortic isthmus shows tubular hypoplasia. In this form the ductus often remains patent, and a ventricular septal defect frequently coexists. Pulmonary hypertension is common. This form has also been called infantile coarctation, because it commonly causes congestive cardiac failure in infancy. (2) Localized coarctation. In this form the ductus is usually closed and coexistent cardiac anomalies are uncommon. When severe, this form leads to failure in infancy. It is the form most commonly found in older patients.

Two anatomic changes occur in response to the coarctation of the aorta: (1) Development of arterial collaterals from the area of high arterial pressure above the coarctation to low arterial pressure below the coarctation. These collaterals involve the intercostals, internal mammary, intraspinal, and scapular arteries. Proximal to the obstruction, blood flows normally into the arteries, but beyond the obstruction, the flow occurs in a retrograde direction into the descending aorta. These collaterals tend to lower aortic pressure proximal to the coarctation and increase perfusion to the lower portion of the body. (2) Development of left ventricular hypertrophy. Left ventricular dilatation may eventually occur.

Hemodynamics. The blood pressure, particularly systolic, is elevated proximally to the coarctation and decreased distally (Fig. 7–10). This difference in blood pressure is the cardinal clinical finding of coarctation of the aorta. The reasons for the hypertension proximal to the coarctation are unknown.

If the coarctation coexists with a ventricular septal defect, the shunt through the defect is increased because of the augmented resistance to left ventricular outflow. This increased resistance is generally compensated for by left ventricular hypertrophy, but in the neonate left ventricular dilatation and failure may occur.

Clinical Features. As indicated, the major finding is differential blood pressure readings between arms and legs. There is commonly a systolic ejection murmur from the flow through the coarctation site. If coexistent conditions are present, additional murmurs are present as well.

In older patients the electrocardiogram is normal, or shows a pattern of left ventricular hypertrophy. In neonates the electrocardiogram typically shows right ventricular hypertrophy and inverted T waves in the left precordial leads.

Echocardiographic Features. M-mode echocardiograms will demonstrate the degree of left ventricular hypertrophy and the presence of major intracardiac anomalies. In neonates the right ventricle is dilated. Two-dimensional echocar-

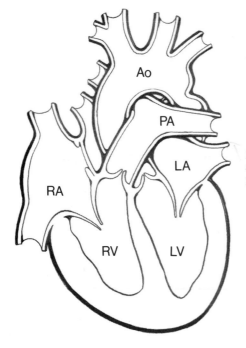

FIGURE 7–10. The central circulation in coarctation of the aorta. Ao, Aorta; LA, left atrium; LV, left ventricle; PA, pulmonary artery; RA, right atrium; RV, right ventricle.

diography, however, allows visualization of the aortic arch—showing the aortic isthmus, the coarctation, and the ductus (Fig. 7–11).

Radiographic Features. Two radiographic pictures exist.

1. Symptomatic infant.
   a. Generalized cardiomegaly (Fig. 7–12).
   b. The pulmonary vasculature shows increased pulmonary venous and arterial vasculature, since there is generally a coexistent ventricular septal defect and congestive cardiac failure.
2. Asymptomatic infant or child.
   a. Normal cardiac size
   b. A prominent left cardiac border from the left ventricular hypertrophy.
   c. Normal pulmonary vascularity.

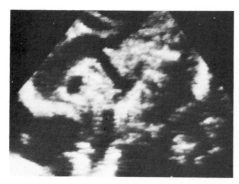
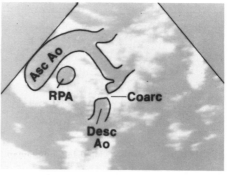

FIGURE 7–11. Coarctation of the aorta. Cross-sectional echocardiogram. Suprasternal view. Coarctation in the proximal descending aorta beyond the left subclavian artery. Coarc, coarctation of aorta; Asc Ao, ascending aorta; Desc Ao, descending aorta; RPA, right pulmonary artery.

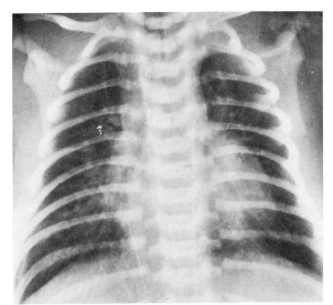

FIGURE 7–12. Coarctation of the aorta in infancy. Prominent, indistinct vascular markings. Cardiomegaly.

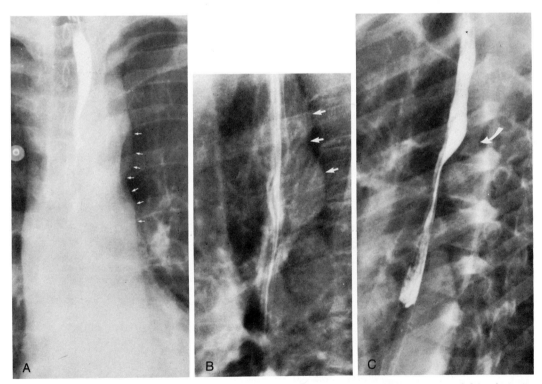

FIGURE 7–13. Coarctation of the aorta. *A,* Figure 3 sign produced by projection of the soft tissues against the lung (arrows). The upper segment is produced by the aortic knob and the dilated left subclavian artery, the waist by the site of coarctation, and the lower segment by the post-stenotic dilatation of the descending aorta. *B,* Lateral chest radiograph with barium swallow: 3 sign produced by projection of the soft tissues against the lung (arrows). The upper part represents the aortic knob and the dilated left subclavian artery, the waist represents the area of coarctation, and the lower part represents the dilated descending aorta beyond the area of coarctation. *C,* Left anterior oblique projection reveals a posterior indentation on the barium-filled esophagus produced by post-stenotic dilatation of the descending aorta pressing against the posterior wall of the esophagus. Note area of coarctation (arrow) and dilated subclavian artery.

d. Post-stenotic dilatation of the proximal descending aorta immediately beyond the coarctation causes a figure **3** or letter **E** configuration. The proximal part is formed medially by the distal aortic arch, and laterally by the dilated proximal left subclavian artery. The distal part is formed by the post-stenotic dilatation of the aorta beyond the coarctation (Figs. 7–13 and 7–14).

e. The aortic knob is not prominent, particularly if tubular hypoplasia coexists (Fig. 7–13).

f. Notching of the inferior margins of the posterior portions of the fourth to eighth ribs is found in older children (beyond 8 years of age) or adults (see Fig. 4–12).

Angiographic Appearance. Aortography is the method of choice to establish the diagnosis of coarctation of the aorta. A lateral or left anterior oblique projection demonstrates the localized, posterior narrowing of the aorta, usually beyond the left subclavian artery. Frequently, hypoplasia of the aortic isthmus coexists (Fig. 7–15). There is an extensive collateral arterial system involving the intercostal, internal mammary, and other thoracic arteries about the coarctation. In infants, balloon occlusion aortography can be performed by passing a balloon catheter through a patent ductus arteriosus into the descending aorta, and injecting proximally to the inflated balloon (Fig. 7–16).

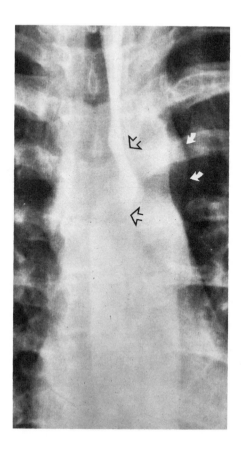

FIGURE 7–14. Coarctation of the aorta. Barium swallow reveals two indentations in the esophagus. The upper indentation is produced by the aortic arch, the lower indentation by the post-stenotic dilatation of the descending aorta (open arrows), producing a "reversed 3 sign." Upper part of the **3** sign (small arrows) is produced by the dilated left subclavian artery and the lower part by the post-stenotic dilatation of the descending aorta.

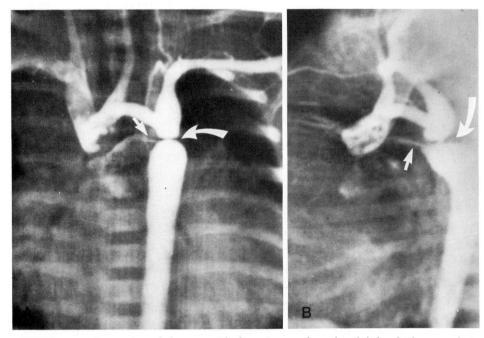

FIGURE 7–15. Coarctation of the aorta. Flush aortogram through a left brachial approach in anteroposterior (A) and lateral (B) projections. Severe coarctation (large arrow) in the aortic isthmus, proximal to the ductus arteriosus (small arrow). Tubular hypoplasia of the aortic arch. Post-stenotic dilatation of the descending aorta.

Management. Coarctation of the aorta is operatively repaired at one of three age periods. (1) One to two months of age, if there is congestive cardiac failure. (2) Three years of age, if there is significant hypertension. (3) Five to six years of age, if the patient is asymptomatic.

One of three operations is performed, depending upon the anatomic data and preference of the surgeon. (1) Resection of coarctation of the aorta and end-to-end anastomosis. (2) Patch angioplasty. A longitudinal incision is made across the coarctation, and a synthetic patch is sewn to widen the coarcted area. (3) Subclavian flap. An incision is made in the descending aorta across the coarctation site; the subclavian artery is divided and opened longitudinally, forming a flap; the flap is then folded downward across the coarcted site into the descending aorta and sewn to widen this portion of the aorta.

FIGURE 7–16. Coarctation of the aorta. *A,* Injection in pulmonary artery: Coarctation faintly seen (arrow). *B,* Balloon occlusion aortogram. Severe coarctation of the aorta proximal to a patent ductus arteriosus (arrow). Ac, Transverse arch; PA, pulmonary artery; Bn, inflated balloon.

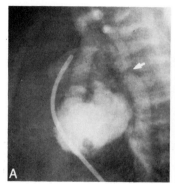
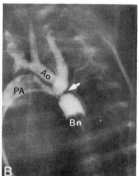

Selected Bibliography

Becker, A. E., Becker, M. J., and Edwards, J. E.: Anomalies associated with coarctation of aorta: Particular reference to infancy. Circulation, *41*:1067–1075, 1970.

Garman, J. G., Hinson, R. E., and Eyler, W. R.: Coarctation of the aorta in infancy: Detection on chest radiographs. Radiology, *85*:418–422, 1965.

Glancy, D. L., Morrow, A. G., Simon, A. L., and Roberts, W. C.: Juxtaductal aortic coarctation: Analysis of 84 patients studied hemodynamically, angiographically, and morphologically after age 1 year. Am. J. Cardiol., *51*:537–551, 1983.

Lock, J. E., Bass, J. L., Amplatz, K., Fuhrman, B. P., and Castaneda-Zuniga, W.: Balloon dilation angioplasty of aortic coarctations in infants and children. Circulation, *68*(1):109–116, 1983.

Smallhorn, J. F., Huhta, J. C., Adams, P. A., Anderson, R. H., Wilkinson, J. L., and Macartney, F. J.: Cross-sectional echocardiographic assessment of coarctation in the sick neonate and infant. Br. Heart J., *50*:349–361, 1983.

Smyth, P. T., and Edwards, J. E.: Pseudocoarctation, kinking or buckling of the aorta. Circulation, *46*:1027–1032, 1972.

INTERRUPTION OF THE AORTIC ARCH

Many features of interruption of aortic arch resemble those of coarctation of the aorta with hypoplasia of the aorta isthmus. In interruption of the aortic arch, the ascending aorta ends blindly beyond either the left carotid artery or the left subclavian artery, while the descending aorta is connected to the pulmonary artery by way of a patent ductus arteriosus (Fig. 7–17). A large ventricular septal defect and often subaortic stenosis coexist. Because of pulmonary hypertension, blood flows from right to left through the ductus arteriosus to supply the lower part of the body. Patients become symptomatic as the ductus arteriosus closes in the neonatal period.

The clinical and radiographic features are identical to coexistent coarctation of the aorta and ventricular septal defect.

Management. This condition is usually corrected in two steps: (1) in infancy

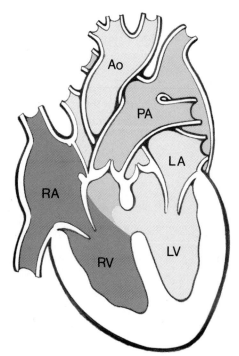

FIGURE 7–17. The central circulation in interruption of the aortic arch between the left carotid and left subclavian arteries. Coexistent ventricular septal defect with left-to-right shunt. Patent ductus arteriosus connecting the pulmonary artery to the descending aorta. Ao, Aorta; LA, left atrium; LV, left ventricle; PA, pulmonary artery; RA, right atrium; RV, right ventricle.

a tube graft is placed between the ascending and descending aorta, and the pulmonary artery banded; (2) around one year of age, the band is removed and the ventricular septal defect closed.

Selected Bibliography

Moller, J. H., and Edwards, J. E.: Interruption of aortic arch: Anatomic patterns and associated cardiac malformations. Am. J. Roentgenol. *95*(3):557–572, 1965.
Riggs, T. W., Berry, T. E., Aziz, K. U., and Paul, M. H.: Two-dimensional echocardiographic features of interruption of the aortic arch. Am. J. Cardiol., *50*:1385–1390, 1982.

PULMONARY STENOSIS

Obstruction to the right ventricular outflow tract may exist with either an intact ventricular septum or a ventricular septal defect. The former is discussed in this chapter; the latter was discussed as tetralogy of Fallot because the clinical and radiographic features are so different. Pulmonary stenosis with intact ventricular septum accounts for 8 per cent of cases of congenital heart disease.

While obstructive lesions may exist at various sites in the right ventricular outflow area, most instances occur at the valve. Peripheral pulmonary arterial stenosis accounts for 5 per cent of pulmonary stenosis with an intact ventricular septum. Isolated infundibular stenosis is rare.

Valvular Pulmonary Stenosis   *c̄ intact septum*

Two anatomic types of valvular pulmonary stenosis exist (Fig. 7–18).

1. Classic (dome-shaped). In this type, which accounts for 95 per cent of all cases of valvular pulmonary stenosis, commissural fusion is present. The stenotic

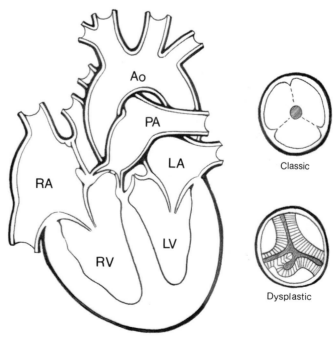

FIGURE 7–18. The central circulation and types of stenotic valves in pulmonary stenosis. Ao, Aorta; LA, left atrium; LV, left ventricle; PA, pulmonary artery; RA, right atrium; RV, right ventricle.

Classic

Dysplastic

valve has a small central orifice and 3 raphes, which represent the fused commissures. The valve tissue is relatively thin and mobile.

2. Dysplastic pulmonary valve. In this type the commissures are not fused. Stenosis occurs because the valve leaflets are thickened, redundant, and immobile; the pulmonary annulus is often hypoplastic.

Hemodynamics. Because of the narrowed pulmonary valvular orifice, the right ventricular systolic pressure rises proportionally to the degree of stenosis.

The right ventricular responds to the increase in right ventricular systolic pressure by development of hypertrophy and not by dilatation.

Pulmonary stenosis progresses with time, because of the development of infundibular stenosis or myocardial fibrosis or both, over decades. Ultimately, right ventricular failure may develop. In patients with elevated right atrial pressure or volume, the foramen ovale may be stretched open, leading to an atrial right-to-left shunt.

Clinical Features. Most patients with pulmonary stenosis are asymptomatic. A few with severe stenosis present with cyanosis or heart failure in infancy. Patients with the dysplastic form are short, have a peculiar facies, and may have a family history of pulmonary stenosis.

There is a loud, pulmonary systolic ejection murmur that transmits to the left back. Often a thrill is associated. A pulmonary systolic ejection click reflecting post-stenotic dilatation is present, except in patients with a dysplastic pulmonary valve.

The electrocardiogram correlates roughly with the severity of the stenosis; with increasing degrees of stenosis, there is more right-axis deviation and right ventricular hypertrophy. Tall P waves, reflecting right atrial hypertrophy, are found in half of the patients. In patients with a dysplastic valve, the QRS axis is usually between 60 and 120 degrees.

Echocardiographic Features. The right ventricular free wall is thickened, and right ventricular internal dimensions are increased. Paradoxical septal motion may be present in patients with a dilated right ventricle. The "a" wave movement of the pulmonary valve is excessive, reflecting the decreased right ventricular compliance. The pulmonary cusps may appear thickened and limited in movement, when viewed on a short-axis, cross-sectional echocardiographic recording (Fig. 7–19).

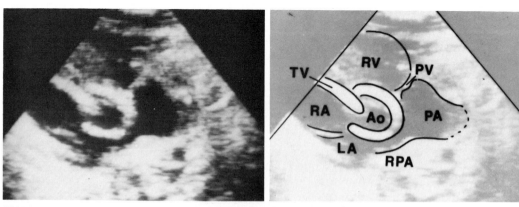

FIGURE 7–19. Pulmonary valvular stenosis. Cross-sectional echocardiogram. Short-axis view. A, Diastole. Both aortic (Ao) and pulmonary (PV) valves closed. B, Systole. Aortic (Ao) valve open. Stenotic pulmonary valve (PV) still appears closed. TV, Tricuspid valve; RV, right ventricle; PV, pulmonary valve; RA, right atrium; Ao, aorta; PA, pulmonary artery; LA, left atrium; RPA, right pulmonary artery.

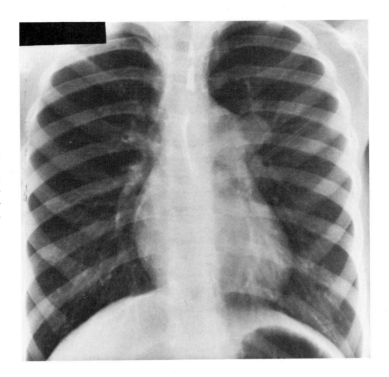

FIGURE 7–20. Pulmonary valvular stenosis. Normal pulmonary arterial vascularity. Normal cardiac size. Prominent pulmonary artery segment with dilatation of the left pulmonary artery. Left aortic arch.

Radiographic Features. The radiographic findings for classic pulmonary stenosis are often diagnostic. There is normal pulmonary vascularity and normal cardiac size, but the pulmonary artery segment and left pulmonary artery are enlarged. This results from post-stenotic dilatation, since the jet of blood through the orifice of the stenotic valve is directed into the left pulmonary artery (Fig. 7–20).

Idiopathic dilatation of the pulmonary artery can be found and it will have

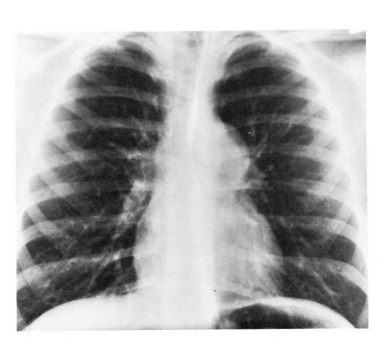

FIGURE 7–21. Idiopathic dilatation of the pulmonary artery. Normal pulmonary arterial vascularity. Normal cardiac size. Marked dilatation of pulmonary artery segment.

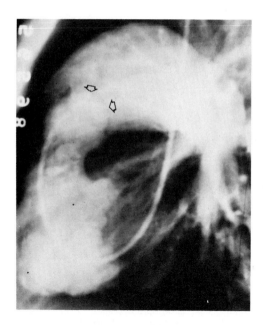

FIGURE 7–22. The same patient as in Figure 7–21. Right ventriculogram in lateral projection. Doming (arrows) of the pulmonary valve. Marked dilatation of the pulmonary artery.

similar radiographic findings (Fig. 7–21). In these cases, a small gradient across the pulmonary valve can be found during catheterization (Fig. 7–22).

In a pulmonary dysplastic valve, pulmonary vascularity, cardiac size, and the cardiac contour are all normal. Thus, the radiographic appearance is usually indistinguishable from normal. There is no post-stenotic dilatation, since a jet is not formed.

Symptomatic Infants

In these patients, pulmonary vascularity is normal unless a right-to-left atrial shunt is present, in which case the vascularity is diminished. The heart is enlarged, often greatly, and has a prominent right (because of the dilated right atrium) and

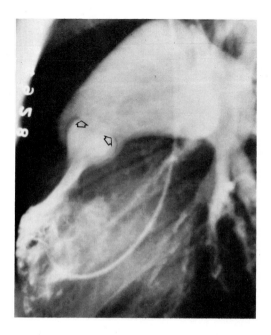

FIGURE 7–23. Pulmonary valvular stenosis. Right ventriculogram in lateral projection. Normal sized right ventricle. Nonobstructed infundibulum. Thin, doming pulmonary valve (arrows). Post-stenotic dilatation of main pulmonary artery.

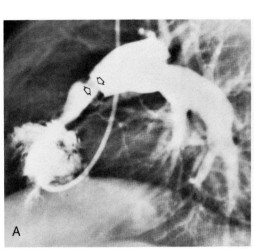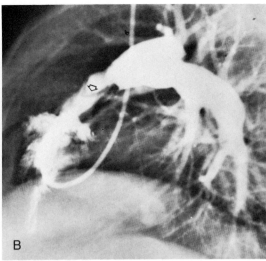

FIGURE 7–24. Pulmonary valvular stenosis. *A,* Systole. Trabeculated right ventricle. Nonobstructed infundibulum. Thickened pulmonary valve (arrows). Blunting of sinuses of Valsalva. Dilatation of main pulmonary artery extending into left pulmonary artery. *B,* Diastole. Thickened pulmonary valve (arrow). Valve appearance changes little between phases of cardiac cycle.

left (because of the dilated right ventricle) border. The pulmonary arterial segment is not dilated. In all forms, the retrosternal space is obliterated in the lateral projection by the hypertrophied right ventricle.

Angiographic Appearance. There are two angiographic appearances of a stenotic pulmonary valve. In classic pulmonary valvular stenosis, the leaflets dome during systole, and a jet of contrast material passes through the center of the valve. The leaflets are thin and freely movable; the main pulmonary artery and left pulmonary artery are dilated, often greatly (Fig. 7–23). In the dysplastic valve, the leaflets are markedly thickened, and their appearance changes little between systole and diastole. There is no central jet and no post-stenotic dilatation (Fig. 7–24).

Management. Patients with symptoms, or asymptomatic patients with a right ventricular systolic pressure greater than 70 mm Hg, should undergo pulmonary valvotomy. In patients with a dysplastic pulmonary valve, one or two cusps are excised, and occasionally a patch is placed across the pulmonary annulus.

Pulmonary insufficiency is present postoperatively but is well tolerated because the pulmonary arterial pressure is low.

Peripheral Pulmonary Arterial Stenosis

Peripheral pulmonary arterial stenosis usually occurs as multiple fusiform narrowings of the major pulmonary arteries in both lungs. The obstruction is usually slight but may be severe enough to raise the right ventricular systolic pressure to 200 mm Hg. Right ventricular hypertrophy results. The condition occurs as a consequence of maternal rubella. It is also present in some children with supravalvular aortic stenosis. A small degree of peripheral pulmonary arterial stenosis is often present in normal premature infants but disappears with growth.

The diagnosis is made clinically by the finding of a systolic ejection murmur heard throughout both lung fields. There is no systolic ejection click. The electrocardiogram is indistinguishable from that seen in valvular pulmonary stenosis.

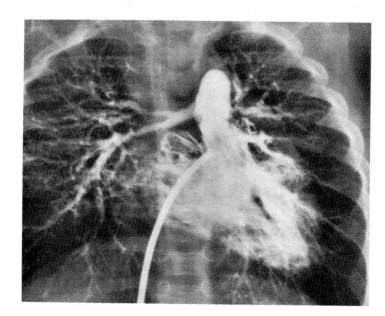

FIGURE 7–25. Peripheral pulmonary artery stenosis. Diffuse hypoplasia of right pulmonary artery. Branches to right upper and lower lobes involved.

Radiographic Features. Pulmonary vascularity is generally normal, although there may be questionable areas of hypovascularity. Cardiac size and contour are normal.

Angiographic Appearance (Fig. 7–25). Single or multiple areas of tubular narrowing can be seen in the proximal right or left pulmonary arteries, or in their major branches. Slight dilatation occurs beyond the narrowed areas.

Management. As a rule, peripheral pulmonary arterial stenosis does not require treatment. When it does, the operation is difficult; the stenotic areas are often multiple, occur at the pulmonary hilus or beyond, and involve small arteries. Balloon dilatation offers a useful form of therapy for these patients.

Selected Bibliography

Castaneda-Zuniga, W. R., Formanek, A., and Amplatz, K.: Radiologic diagnosis of different types of pulmonary stenoses. Cardiovasc. Radiol., *1*:45–57, 1978.

Johnson, L. W., Grossman, W., Dalen, J. E., and Dexter, L.: Pulmonic stenosis in the adult: Long-term follow-up results. N. Engl. J. Med., *287*(23):1159–1198, 1972.

Lucas, R. V., and Moller, J. H.: Pulmonary valvular stenosis. Cardiovasc. Clin., *2*(1):156–184, 1967.

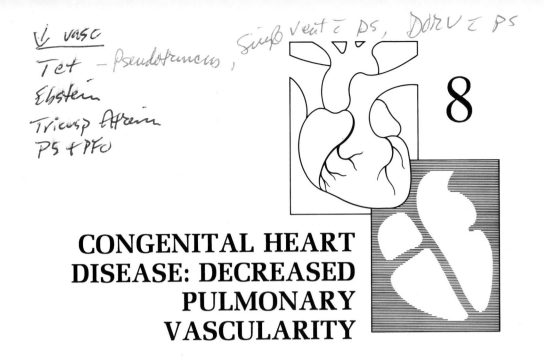

8

CONGENITAL HEART DISEASE: DECREASED PULMONARY VASCULARITY

Several cardiac conditiona are associated with decreased pulmonary vascularity. In each, there is obstruction of the pulmonary blood flow and an intracardiac defect, through which blood is shunted away from the lungs toward the body, causing cyanosis. The intracardiac defect may be located at either the ventricular or the atrial level. Cardiac size is usually normal in the former situation and increased in the latter.

Normal Cardiac Size

In most patients with cyanosis, decreased pulmonary vascularity, and normal cardiac size, tetralogy of Fallot is the underlying cardiac condition.

Tetralogy of Fallot

Tetralogy of Fallot represents 8 per cent of congenital heart disease. As the name indicates, the malformation has four components (Fig. 8–1).

1. A ventricular septal defect, which is large and located immediately below the aortic valve.

2. A pulmonary stenosis, which is usually located in the infundibulum and is caused by either hypoplasia or hypertrophy of the crista supraventricularis. The pulmonary annulus and arterial tree may be hypoplastic and the pulmonary valve stenotic.

3. An overriding aorta, which straddles the ventricular septal defect to a variable extent or which causes the vessel to receive blood from both ventricles.

4. A right ventricular hypertrophy, which occurs as a result of the elevated right ventricular systolic pressure.

Hemodynamics. Because the ventricular septal defect is large, the right ventricular systolic pressure is elevated, being equal to the left ventricular and aortic systolic pressures. The direction and magnitude of blood flow through the

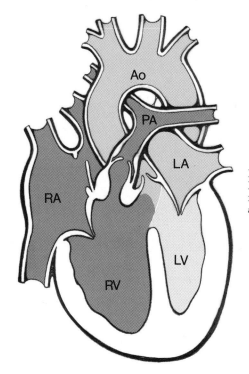

FIGURE 8–1. The central circulation in tetralogy of Fallot. Right-to-left shunt at ventricular level. Ao, Aorta; PA, pulmonary artery; LA, left atrium; LV, left ventricle; RA, right atrium; RV, right ventricle.

defect depend on the relative resistances imposed by the pulmonary stenosis and the systemic vascular bed. In tetralogy of Fallot, pulmonary stenosis offers more resistance, and a right-to-left shunt occurs through the defect (Fig. 8–1). Any event, such as exercise, that lowers systemic vascular resistance or that increases infundibular pulmonary stenosis, such as beta-catecholamine stimulation, causes a larger shunt.

Clinical Features. The clinical history of a patient with tetralogy of Fallot is frequently diagnostic. The degree of cyanosis is extremely variable and often changes rapidly. Hot weather, meals, and exercise typically increase cyanosis because each lowers the systemic vascular resistance.

"Tetrad spells" occur in many infants and young children. These characteristic episodes are associated with a sudden marked increase in the right-to-left shunt leading to severe hypoxemia. The arterial pO_2 may drop as low as 10 mm Hg. Early symptoms of a spell include restlessness, followed by listlessness. Coma, convulsions, and death may ensue. These may occur during a cardiac catheterization. Another characteristic symptom is squatting. As the child exercises and becomes tired, he assumes a squatting position, which increases the systemic vascular resistance, decreases the right-to-left shunt, and lessens the cyanosis. Congestive cardiac failure does not occur. Growth and motor development may be delayed, but language and other features of mental development are normal.

The principal auscultatory finding is a pulmonary systolic ejection murmur, which results from blood flow through the pulmonary stenosis and not through the ventricular septal defect. The loudness of the murmur is inversely related to the severity of the stenosis.

The electrocardiogram shows right-axis deviation (usually between +120 and +150 degrees) and right ventricular hypertrophy, usually with an rR' pattern in lead V_1.

Echocardiographic Features. The echocardiogram is usually diagnostic. It

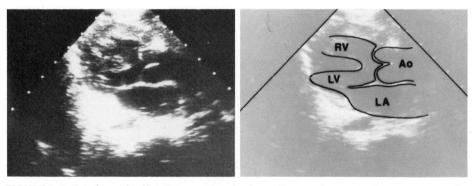

FIGURE 8–2. Tetralogy of Fallot. Cross-sectional echocardiogram. Long-axis view. Aorta overrides ventricular septal defect. RV, Right ventricle; AO, aorta; LV, left ventricle; LA, left atrium.

shows a deficiency in the ventricular septum immediately below the aortic valve. The anterior wall of the aorta is not in continuity and lies anteriorly to the interventricular septum, indicating the aortic overriding (Fig. 8–2). Usually the narrowed pulmonary annulus can be seen. The free right ventricular wall is thickened, and the right ventricular internal dimensions may be increased. In contrast to the findings in most patients with truncus arteriosus, the left atrial and left ventricular dimensions are normal. From the suprasternal notch, the dilated ascending aorta may be visualized and compared with the size of the pulmonary arteries (Fig. 8–3).

    Radiographic Features. The chest radiograph is often typical. The pulmonary arterial vascularity is decreased, because pulmonary blood flow is limited by the stenosis (Fig. 8–4), although in less severe cases it may appear normal (Fig. 8–5). A bizarre vascular pattern can be seen in the presence of large bronchial collaterals (Fig. 8–6). Normal pulmonary vascular markings with a history of cyanosis usually suggest tetralogy of Fallot. Cardiac size is normal, but the cardiac contour is abnormal and has been described as boot-shaped (Figs. 8–4 to 8–6). This contour results from several features. The aorta is enlarged and the pulmonary arterial segment concave. Because of the right ventricular hypertrophy, the cardiac apex is elevated and rounded. In one fourth of cases, the aortic arch is right-sided.

    Angiographic Appearance. Right ventriculography obtained in anteroposterior and lateral projections provides adequate demonstration of the anatomic details of the anomaly. After injection of contrast material into the right ventricle, the aorta opacifies because of the right-to-left shunt. The overriding of the aorta

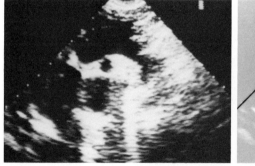
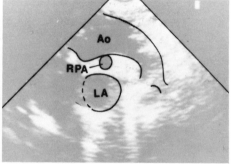

FIGURE 8–3. Tetralogy of Fallot. Cross-sectional echocardiogram. Suprasternal notch view. Enlarged aorta and tiny right pulmonary artery (RPA). Ao, Aorta; LA, left atrium.

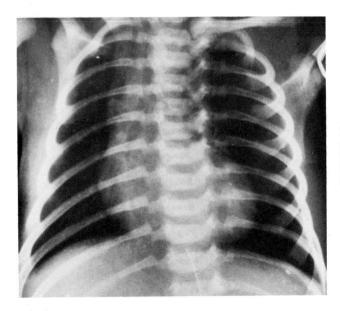

FIGURE 8–4. Tetralogy of Fallot. Decreased pulmonary arterial vascularity. Normal cardiac size. Round cardiac apex. Concave pulmonary segment. Right aortic arch.

and the narrowing of the right ventricular outflow tract is best demonstrated in a slight right anterior oblique projection by a vertical x-ray tube (Fig. 8–7).

The pulmonary valve is frequently bicuspid and shows a characteristic "clamshell" deformity in a lateral projection (Fig. 8–8). The pulmonary arteries are frequently hypoplastic.

Left ventriculography in a long-axial-like projection demonstrates well the position and number of ventricular septal defects and the overriding of the aortic root. Size and contractility of the left ventricle can be assessed from the vertical plane of the long-axial oblique projection.

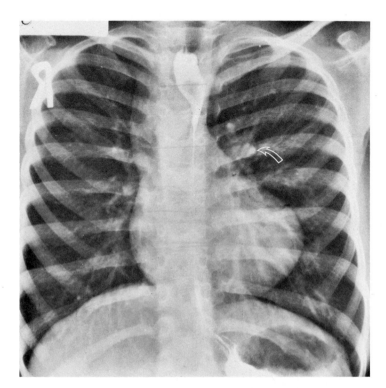

FIGURE 8–5. Tetralogy of Fallot. Normal pulmonary arterial vascularity. Unusual vascular markings in the left lung from large systemic collaterals (open arrow). Normal cardiac size. Round uplifted apex causes a boot-shaped configuration. Right aortic arch.

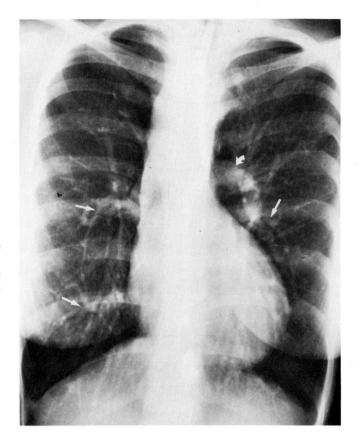

FIGURE 8–6. Tetralogy of Fallot. Abnormal appearance of the pulmonary arterial vascularity in both lung fields, more on right, from large systemic collaterals to both upper and the right lower lobes (straight arrows). Comma-like appearance of left pulmonary artery, frequently present in tetralogy of Fallot (curved arrow). Normal cardiac size. Round uptilted apex. Concave pulmonary artery segment. Right aortic arch.

An aortogram should be performed in a shallow left anterior oblique projection to study the anatomy of the coronary arteries. In 10 per cent of cases, the left anterior descending artery arises from the right coronary artery and passes across the anterior outflow tract of the right ventricle.

Management. Two types of operations are available: palliative and corrective.

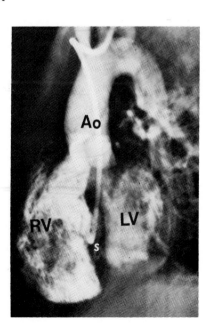

FIGURE 8–7. Tetralogy of Fallot. Right ventriculogram in lateral projection. Aorta (Ao) overrides the ventricular septum (S). Opacification of left ventricle (LV) through ventricular septal defect. RV, Right ventricle.

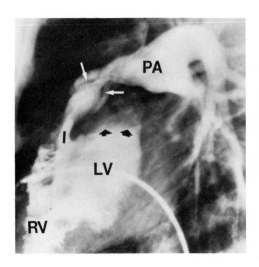

FIGURE 8–8. Tetralogy of Fallot. Right ventriculogram in lateral projection. Contrast medium passes through the ventricular septal defect into the left ventricle (LV). Narrowed infundibulum. "Clamshell" appearance of a doming bicuspid valve (white arrows). RV, Right ventricle; I, infundibulum; PA, pulmonary artery. Aortic valve (black arrows).

The four palliative operations are used in symptomatic infants or patients with small or hypoplastic pulmonary arteries.

1. Potts procedure. A communication is created between the left pulmonary artery and the descending aorta to permit blood flow from the aorta to the pulmonary circulation. The Potts procedure has been largely abandoned.

2. Waterston procedure. A communication is made between the ascending aorta and the right pulmonary artery.

3. Central shunt. A tubular synthetic graft is inserted between the ascending aorta and the pulmonary artery. This is generally the preferred palliative procedure for infants.

4. Blalock-Taussig operation. The subclavian artery on the side opposite the aortic arch is divided and anastomosed to the ipsilateral pulmonary artery. This shunt allows a portion of the blood reaching the aorta to enter the pulmonary artery and become oxygenated. This is generally the preferred operation for older children requiring palliation.

A corrective operation involves the closing of the ventricular septal defect and the alleviation of the right ventricular outflow obstruction, usually by a combination of pulmonary valvotomy, resection of infundibular myocardium, and placement of an outflow patch to widen the hypoplastic outflow area. The operation can be performed electively in children or in symptomatic infants, provided that the pulmonary arteries are large enough.

Tetralogy of Fallot with Pulmonary Atresia (Pseudotruncus)

In this condition, the anatomic features of tetralogy of Fallot are present, but the pulmonary valve is atretic. Pulmonary blood flow is derived either from a patent ductus arteriosus (Fig. 8–9) or from systemic collateral arteries 'Fig. 8–10) that arise from the descending aorta and connect with the pulmonary arterial tree at the hilus or at a more peripheral site in the pulmonary arterial tree. The size, number, and origin of these vessels vary considerably. When the pulmonary blood flow depends principally on the ductus arteriosus, severe signs and symptoms appear in the neonatal period when the ductus closes. On the other hand, cyanosis may be minimal in the occasional patient with large and multiple systemic collaterals.

The unique physical finding of this condition is a continuous murmur either

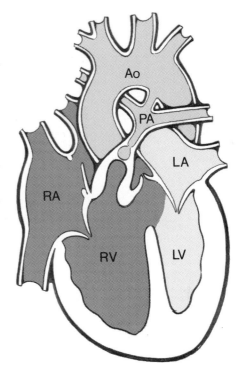

FIGURE 8–9. The central circulation in tetralogy of Fallot with pulmonary atresia. Patent ductus arteriosus provides source of pulmonary blood flow. Ao, Aorta; LA, left atrium; LV, left ventricle; PA, pulmonary artery; RA, right atrium; RV, right ventricle.

from the ductus arteriosus or from the systemic collateral arteries. The electrocardiogram, showing a right-axis deviation and a right ventricular hypertrophy, is indistinguishable from that seen in tetralogy of Fallot. The echocardiogram also resembles that of tetralogy of Fallot in showing a ventricular septal defect and an

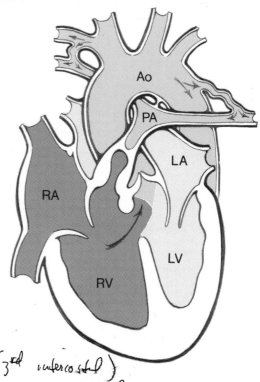

FIGURE 8–10. The central circulation in tetralogy of Fallot with pulmonary atresia and bronchial collateral arteries to pulmonary arteries. Right-to-left shunt at ventricular level. Abbreviations as in Figure 8–9.

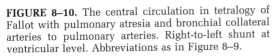

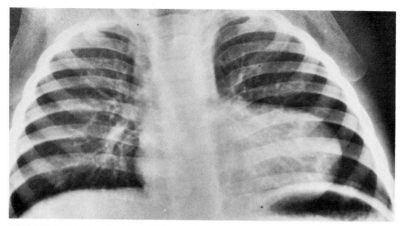

FIGURE 8–11. Tetralogy of Fallot with pulmonary atresia. Asymmetry of pulmonary vascular markings, more prominent in the right lung. Cardiomegaly with a boot-shaped configuration. Concave pulmonary artery segment. Left aortic arch.

overriding aorta, but a pulmonary valve and a pulmonary artery cannot be demonstrated. However, failure to demonstrate the pulmonary valve and artery is not diagnostic, because the failure may result from technical problems with the echocardiographic recording.

Radiographic Features. Cardiomegaly may be present if the volume of pulmonary blood flow is increased (Figs. 8–11 and 8–12). The cardiac contour is boot-shaped, and the aorta is more prominent. The pulmonary vasculature is often bizarre, not showing distinct hila but showing bronchial arteries entering the lungs at unusual sites (Figs. 8–6 and 8–12).

Angiographic Appearance. Right ventriculography demonstrates the presence of a ventricular septal defect, overriding of the aorta, and a blind-ending infundibulum (Figs. 8–13 and 8–14). The pulmonary arteries fill either through a

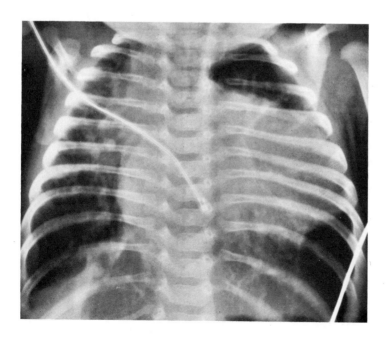

FIGURE 8–12. Tetralogy of Fallot with pulmonary atresia. Prominent hilar vessels. Multiple vascular cross sections indicate large systemic collaterals to lungs. Marked cardiomegaly. Round uplifted apex. Right aortic arch.

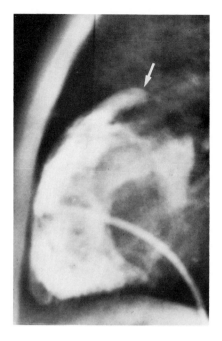

FIGURE 8–13. Tetralogy of Fallot with pulmonary atresia. Right ventriculogram demonstrates a blind ending infundibulum (small arrow).

patent ductus arteriosus or through bronchial arteries that join the pulmonary arteries in the hilum or more distal sites (Figs. 8–14-*B* and 8–15).

Management. These patients, like those with tetralogy of Fallot, often require a palliative shunt. Correction is available in some children by closure of the ventricular septal defect and reconstruction of the right ventricular outflow area, often with a valved conduit.

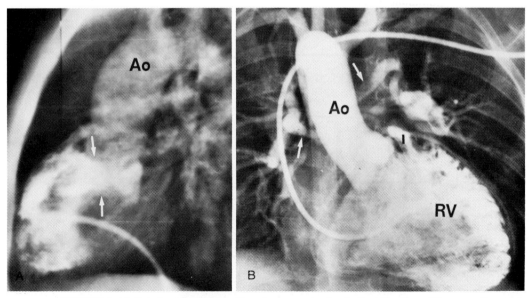

FIGURE 8–14. Tetralogy of Fallot with pulmonary atresia. *A*, Opacification of the ascending aorta through a ventricular septal defect (arrows). Ao, Aorta. *B*, Right aortic arch. Systemic collateral artery (white arrows) from the descending aorta. AO, Aorta; RV, right ventricle; I, blind ending infundibulum.

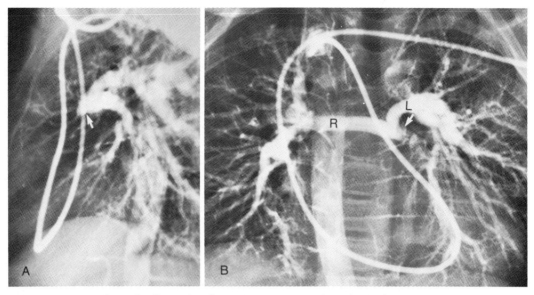

FIGURE 8–15. Tetralogy of Fallot with pulmonary atresia. Late phase descending aortogram. *A*, Anteroposterior, and *B*, lateral projections. Opacification of the left (L) and right (R) pulmonary arteries through systemic collaterals. Small pulmonary artery trunk (arrow).

Tetralogy of Fallot Variants

Other cardiac conditions with pulmonary stenosis and a ventricular communication present hemodynamic, clinical, and radiographic findings similar to those seen in tetralogy of Fallot. These conditions include (1) single ventricle with pulmonary stenosis; (2) double-outlet right ventricle with pulmonary stenosis; (3) transposition, ventricular septal defect, and pulmonary stenosis; (4) atrioventricular canal and pulmonary stenosis; and (5) cardiac conditions associated with the asplenia syndrome.

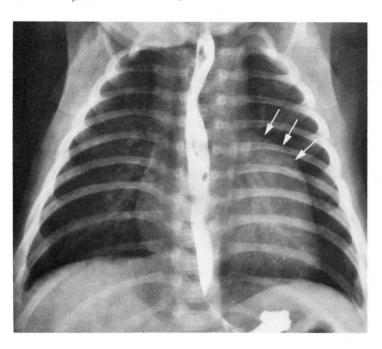

FIGURE 8–16. Single ventricle and levotransposition of great vessels. Normal pulmonary arterial vascularity. Cardiomegaly with a prominent left upper cardiac border (arrows).

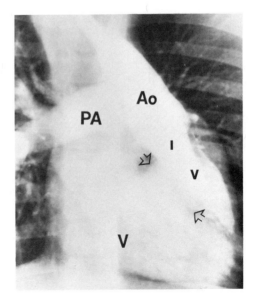

FIGURE 8–17. Single ventricle and levotransposition of great vessels. Ventriculogram in anteroposterior projection. Injection into a small subaortic ventricular chamber (v). Large ventricular communication (arrows) with larger (single) ventricle (V). Pulmonary artery (PA) originates from single ventricle. Aorta (Ao) arises from infundibulum (I) and ascends on left.

Single Ventricle. The plain film radiographic findings can be characteristic, with prominence of the left upper heart border due to the inversion of the right ventricular outflow tract, and to the levoposition of the ascending aorta, which arises from the inverted infundibulum (Figs. 8–16 and 8–17). If there is no pulmonary valve stenosis, pulmonary blood flow can be markedly increased (Fig. 8–18).

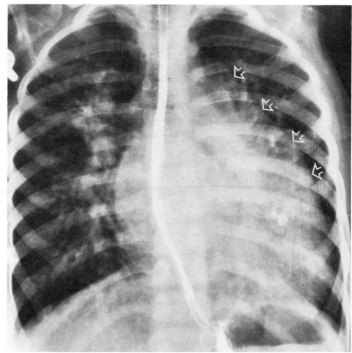

FIGURE 8–18. Single ventricle. Increased pulmonary arterial vascularity. Prominence of the hilar vessels. Cardiomegaly. Prominent left upper cardiac border with vascular shadow extending into mediastinum along the left upper cardiac border represents ascending aorta (open arrows).

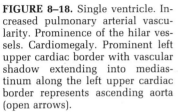

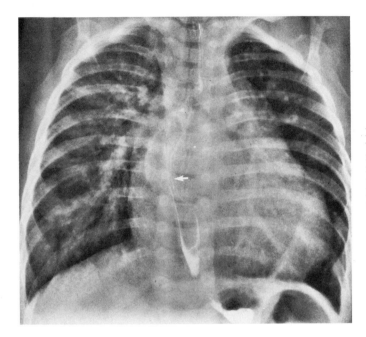

FIGURE 8–19. Double outlet right ventricle. Markedly increased pulmonary arterial vascularity. Cardiomegaly. Enlarged left atrium displaces esophagus to the right (arrow). Prominent pulmonary artery segment. Round upturned cardiac apex.

Double Outlet Right Ventricle. If pulmonary stenosis is present, the pulmonary blood flow will be decreased. The pulmonary segment can be absent, depending on the degree of change in position of the pulmonary artery. In the absence of pulmonary stenosis, the plain film findings can be identical to those of a ventricular septal defect (Figs. 8–19 and 8–20).

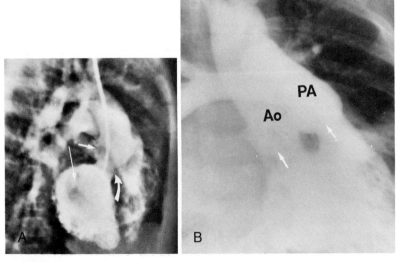

FIGURE 8–20. Right ventriculogram in double outlet right ventricle. *A,* Lateral projection. Aortic valve (short arrow) separated from mitral valve (long arrow). Large ventricular septal defect (curved arrow). *B,* Anteroposterior projection. Semilunar valves positioned at the same level (arrows). Ao, Aorta; PA, pulmonary artery.

Selected Bibliography

Braunlin, E. A., Formanek, A. G., Moller, J. H., and Jesse, E. E.: Angio-pathological appearances of pulmonary valve in pulmonary atresia with intact ventricular septum: Interpretation of nature of right ventricle from pulmonary angiography. Br. Heart J., *47*:281–289, 1981.

Bull, C., DeLeval, M. R., Mercanti, C., Macartney, F. J., and Anderson, R. H.: Pulmonary atresia and intact ventricular septum: A revised classification. Circulation, *66*(2):266–272, 1982.

Formanek, A., Marin-Garcia, J., and Moller, J. H.: Single ventricle: A new angiographic classification. Fortschr. Rontgenstr., *123*(3):210–218, 1975.

Goldsmith, M., Farina, M. A., and Shaher, R. M.: Tetralogy of Fallot with atresia of the left pulmonary artery. J. Thorac., Cardiovasc. Surg., *69*(3):458–466, 1975.

Marin-Garcia, J., Tandon, R., Moller, J. H., and Edwards, J. E.: Common (single) ventricle with normally related great vessels. Circulation, *49*:565–573, 1974.

Neufeld, H. N., Jr., Lester, R. G., Adams, P., Jr., Anderson, R. C., and Edwards, J. E.: Origin of both great vessels from the right ventricle without pulmonary stenosis. Br. Heart J., *24*(4):373–408, 1962.

Partridge, J. B., and Fiddler, G. I.: Cineangiocardiography in tetralogy of Fallot. Br. Heart J., *45*:112–121. 1981.

Sahn, D. J., Harder, J. R., Freedom, R. M., Duncan, W. J., Rowe, R. D., Allen, H. D., Valdes-Cruz, L., and Goldberg, S. J.: Cross-sectional echocardiographic diagnosis and subclassification of univentricular hearts: Imaging studies of atrioventricular valves, septal structures and rudimentary outflow chambers. Circulation, *66*(5):1070–1077, 1982.

Soto, B., Pacifico, A. D., and DiSciascio, G.: Univentricular heart: An angiographic study. Am. J. Cardiol., *49*:787–794, 1982.

Sridaromont, S., Ritter, D. G., Feldt, R. H., Davis, G. D., and Edwards, J. E.: Double-outlet right ventricle: Anatomic and angiocardiographic correlations. Mayo Clin. Proc., *53*:555–577, 1978.

Zamora, R., Moller, J. H., and Edwards, J. E.: Double-outlet right ventricle: Anatomic types and associated anomalies. Chest, *68*:672–677, 1975.

Increased Cardiac Size

In most patients with right ventricular outflow obstruction, with an intact ventricular septum and an atrial right-to-left shunt, cardiomegaly is present. The cardiomegaly results principally from an enlarged right atrium.

Tricuspid Atresia

This congenital cardiac anomaly accounts for 1.5 per cent of all instances of congenital heart disease.

Anatomy and Classification. The tricuspid valve is absent, and the inflow portion of the right ventricle is hypoplastic. The infundibular area of the right ventricle is fairly well developed, but in severe cases with limited pulmonary blood flow, it is slitlike. There is an interatrial communication, leading to right atrial enlargement. In most patients, a ventricular septal defect coexists, but it may be small; pulmonary valvular stenosis or atresia may also coexist.

Tricuspid atresia has been classified into two major groups according to the presence or absence of transposition of the great vessels and pulmonary stenosis.

1. Tricuspid atresia without transposition 80 per cent) (Fig. 8–21)
   a. With pulmonary atresia
   b. With pulmonary stenosis
   c. Without pulmonary stenosis
2. Tricuspid atresia with transposition of the great vessels (Fig. 8–22)
   a. With pulmonary atresia
   b. With pulmonary stenosis
   c. Without pulmonary stenosis

Hemodynamics. Because of the tricuspid valvular obstruction, a right-to-left shunt is created at the atrial level. The left atrium receives the entire systemic and pulmonary venous return, which mixes both there and in the left ventricle. From the left ventricle, blood is ejected into the aorta and, through the ventricular

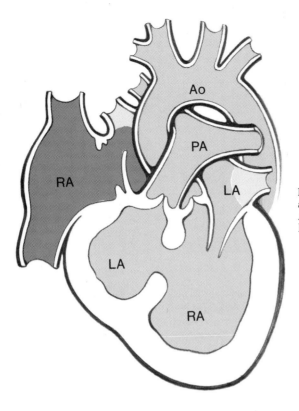

FIGURE 8–21. The central circulation in tricupsid atresia with normally related great vessels. Ao, Aorta; PA, pulmonary artery; LA, left atrium; LV, left ventricle; RA, right atrium; RV, right ventricle.

septal defect, into the pulmonary arteries. The proportional distributions of blood to the lungs and body depend on the resistances to flow. Usually, the sizes of the ventricular septal defect and infundibular chamber, as well as the stenosis of the pulmonary valve, limit the volume of pulmonary blood flow.

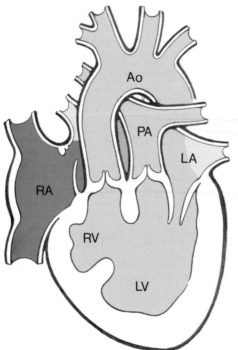

FIGURE 8–22. The central circulation in tricuspid atresia with transposition of the great vessels. Ao, Aorta; PA, pulmonary artery, LA, left atrium; LV, left ventricle; RA, right atrium; RV, right ventricle.

Because there is <u>uniform mixing of the two venous returns,</u> tricuspid atresia is considered an admixture lesion. As in other such lesions, there is an inverse relation between the degree of cyanosis and the volume of pulmonary blood flow; most patients are severely cyanotic. In patients without pulmonary stenosis, particularly those with transposition of the great vessels, the volume of pulmonary blood flow is great and cyanosis minimal. However, these patients develop congestive cardiac failure because of left ventricular volume overload.

Clinical Features. Cyanosis progresses from birth, and its severity is inversely proportional to the volume of pulmonary blood flow. There is a pansystolic murmur along the left sternal border; the loudness of the murmur reflects the volume of flow through the ventricular septal defect.

The electrocardiogram is diagnostic: left-axis deviation, left ventricular hypertrophy, and right atrial enlargement are found. Often, T waves are inverted in the left precordial leads.

Echocardiographic Features. Echocardiographic recordings are not in themselves diagnostic but can strongly support the other clinical and laboratory data. Echoes cannot be recorded from the tricuspid valve. The anterior ventricular cavity (outflow tract of the right ventricle) is small, and the left ventricle is enlarged. The pulmonary valve may be stenotic. Two-dimensional echocardiography also shows these features and, in addition, demonstrates the relations of the great vessels.

Radiographic Features. The typical radiographic features are best seen in posteroanterior and left anterior oblique projections. The cardiac size is variable, ranging from normal to moderately enlarged, and depends on two factors: (1) the volume of pulmonary blood flow, and (2) the right atrial size, which may be increased, particularly if the foramen ovale is restrictive. The cardiac contour is often typical. On a posteroanterior projection, the left border has a characteristic rounded contour because of enlargement and hypertrophy of the left ventricle, while the right cardiac border shows the enlarged convexity of the right atrium. The pulmonary arterial segment is flat or concave. The pulmonary vascularity is normal or decreased (Fig. 8–23). A right aortic arch is uncommon.

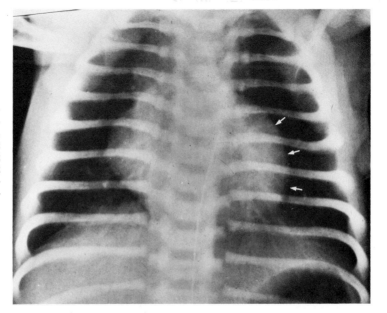

FIGURE 8–23. Tricuspid atresia. Decreased pulmonary arterial vascularity. Cardiomegaly. Prominent right lower cardiac border from enlarged right atrium. Very round prominent left cardiac border from enlargement of left ventricle (arrows).

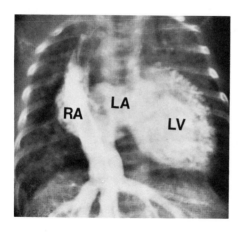

FIGURE 8–24. Tricuspid atresia. Right atriogram in antero-posterior projection. Right-to-left shunt at atrial level. No forward flow from the right atrium into the right ventricle. Left ventricle (LV) opacifies through mitral valve. RA, right atrium; LA, left atrium.

Angiographic Appearance. Angiography usually reveals the absence of communication of the right atrium with the right ventricle (Fig. 8–24). A small smooth depression may be seen at the site of the normal tricuspid valve. An obligatory right-to-left shunt at the atrial level is present. Left ventriculography in axial oblique projections is needed to demonstrate the size and level of the ventricular septal defect.

Management. The type of operative management depends on the decrease or increase of the pulmonary blood flow. When it is decreased, the same palliative procedures used in patients with tetralogy of Fallot are appropriate. When the patient is beyond infancy, a conduit is placed between the right atrium and the pulmonary artery, and the atrial septal defect is closed so that all the systemic venous return is delivered to the pulmonary artery (Fontan procedure). The long-term results of this procedure need to be evaluated. In patients with increased pulmonary blood flow, a pulmonary arterial band can be placed. In these patients, if pulmonary vascular disease does not develop, it may eventually be possible to perform a Fontan procedure.

Selected Bibliography

Rao, P. S.: Fundamentals and clinical cardiology: A unified classification of tricuspid atresia. Am. Heart J., 99(6):799–804, 1980.
Seward, J. B., Tajik, A. J., Hagler, D. J., and Ritter, D. G.: Echocardiographic spectrum of tricuspid atresia. Mayo Clin. Proc., 53:100–112, 1978.
Tandon, R., and Edwards, J. E.: Tricuspid atresia. J. Thorac. Cardiovasc. Surg., 67(4):530–542, 1974.

Ebstein's Malformation of the Tricuspid Valve

This is an infrequently occurring type of congenital heart disease, in which downward displacement of the tricuspid valve occurs. The posterior and septal leaflets originate abnormally from the right ventricular wall, while the anterior leaflet of the tricuspid valve is normal. The displaced leaflets adhere directly to the right ventricular wall or are attached by anomalous chordae tendinae and papillary muscles. The tricuspid valve is often insufficient. The degree of displacement of the tricuspid valve varies considerably. The volume of the right ventricle distal to the tricuspid valve is reduced, while the right atrium is enlarged because of tricuspid insufficiency and by the portion of the ventricle (atrialized portion) proximal to the tricuspid valve. A patent foramen ovale or atrial septal defect is almost always present.

Hemodynamics. The severity of the hemodynamics depends upon the degree

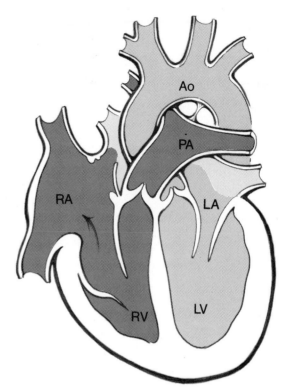

FIGURE 8–25. The central circulation in Ebstein's malformation of the tricuspid valve. Ao, aorta; LA, left atrium; LV, left ventricle; PA, pulmonary artery; RA, right atrium; RV, right ventricle.

of downward displacement of the tricuspid valve. Because of the reduced volume, the functional right ventricular cavity, and the degree of tricuspid insufficiency, the volume of antegrade flow from the right ventricle is reduced. Therefore, right atrial pressure is elevated and a right-to-left shunt occurs at the atrial level through the atrial septal defect (Fig. 8–25).

Clinical Features. Most patients with Ebstein's abnormality present with cyanosis in the neonatal period. This may be associated with congestive cardiac failure. Some patients improve and are essentially asymptomatic for long periods of time. There is a tendency for patients to have episodes of paroxysmal atrial tachycardia. A systolic murmur presents along the left sternal border and is associated with multiple heart sounds.

The electrocardiogram is diagnostic and shows right atrial enlargement and either right bundle-branch block or a pattern of Wolff-Parkinson-White syndrome.

Echocardiographic Features. The M-mode echocardiogram shows a delayed tricuspid valve closure and paradoxical motion of the interventricular septum. The abnormal attachment of the tricuspid valve, the reduced size of the right ventricular cavity, and dilatation of the right atrium can be identified by cross-sectional echocardiography.

Radiographic Features. A thoracic roentgenogram may show striking cardiomegaly and reduced pulmonary vasculature (Fig. 8–26). In some patients the pulmonary vasculature may appear normal, although the films still show cardiomegaly and right atrial enlargement (Fig. 8–27).

Angiographic Features. Angiographic studies, particularly right ventriculograms, are usually diagnostic. Generally there is tricuspid regurgitation following injection into the right ventricle. A diagnosis is made by identification of a notch in the right ventricle that marks the location of the displaced tricuspid valve (Figs.

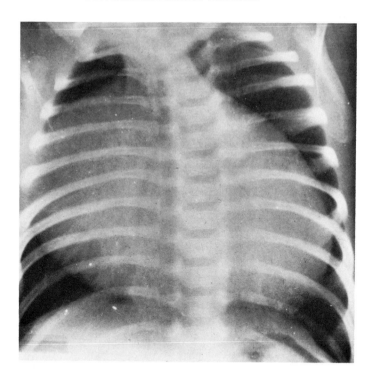

FIGURE 8–26. Ebstein's malformation. Decreased pulmonary arterial vascularity. Massive cardiomegaly. Enlarged right cardiac border suggesting right atrial enlargement. Cardiac apex is displaced downward and laterally.

8–28 and 8–29). Usually the distal part of the right ventricle is reduced in size and empties slowly. In cineangiography the paradoxical motion of the atrialized portion of the right ventricle may be noted. Atrial injections may be misleading because the right-to-left atrial shunt and subsequent opacification of left-sided cardiac chambers can obscure the details of the overlying right ventricular cavity.

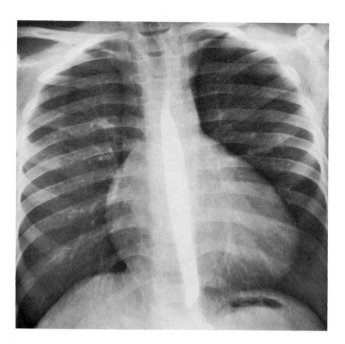

FIGURE 8–27. Ebstein's malformation. Normal pulmonary arterial vascularity. Cardiomegaly. Prominent right cardiac border indicating right atrial enlargement.

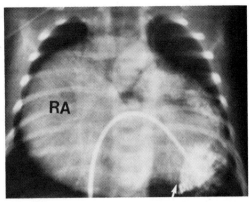

FIGURE 8–28. The same patient as in Figure 8–26. Right ventriculogram in anteroposterior projection. Massive tricuspid insufficiency. Opacification of entire right atrium (RA). Tricuspid valve (arrow) displaced leftward.

Management. Management is generally with digitalis and diuretics in symptomatic patients. In older patients who are symptomatic, placement of a prosthetic tricuspid valve has been performed.

Pulmonary Stenosis in Atrial Septal Defect with Right-to-Left Shunt

This condition must be considered in the differential diagnosis of patients with cyanosis, cardiomegaly, and decreased pulmonary arterial markings (Fig. 8–30). This condition, which occurs primarily in symptomatic infants, was discussed previously in the section on Pulmonary Stenosis (pages 141–146).

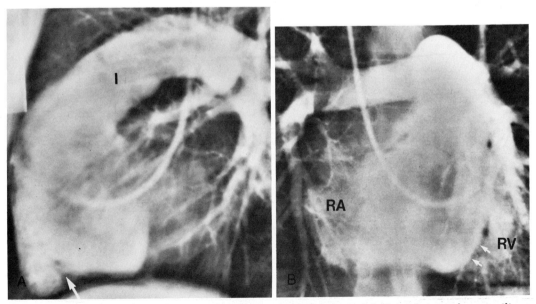

FIGURE 8–29. Ebstein's malformation. A, Lateral right ventriculography reveals a curvilinear radiolucency at the base of the ventricle (arrow) indicating position of downwardly displaced tricuspid valve. Widely open infundibulum (I). B, Anteroposterior projection in right ventriculogram. Downward displacement of the tricuspid valve (arrows). Marked tricuspid reflux is present. RA, Right atrium; RV, right ventricle.

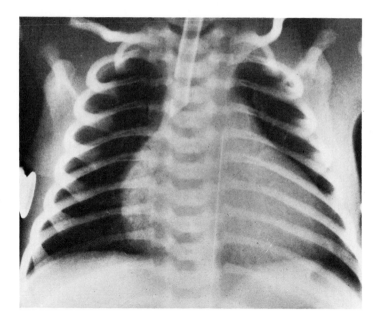

FIGURE 8–30. Decreased pulmonary vascularity and cardiomegaly in a newborn with cyanosis.

Selected Bibliography

Anderson, K. R., Zuberbuhler, J. R., Anderson, R. H., Becker, A. E., and Lie, J. T.: Morphologic spectrum of Ebstein's anomaly of the heart: A review. Mayo Clin. Proc., *54*:174–180, 1979.

Giuliani, E. R., Fuster, V., Brandenberg, R. O., and Mair, D. D.: Ebstein's anomaly: The clinical features and natural history of Ebstein's anomaly of the tricuspid valve. Mayo Clin. Proc., *54*:163–173, 1979.

Shina, A., Seward, J. B., Tajik, A. J., Hagler, D. J., and Danielson, G. K.: Two-dimensional echocardiograph—surgical correlation in Ebstein's anomaly: Preoperative determination of patients requiring tricuspid valve plication vs. replacement. Circulation, *68*(3):534–544, 1983.

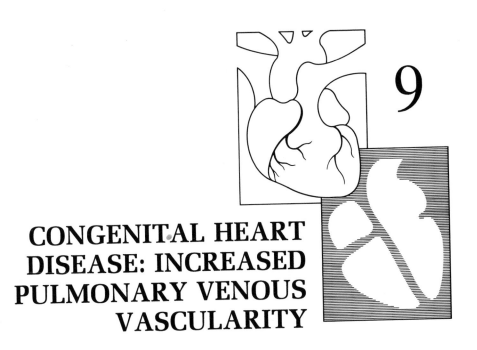

CONGENITAL HEART DISEASE: INCREASED PULMONARY VENOUS VASCULARITY

A variety of cardiac conditions with elevated pulmonary venous pressure shows a radiographic appearance of increased venous vascularity. The conditions may be broadly divided on the basis of whether the cardiac anomaly is located proximally or distally to the mitral valve. If the obstructive lesion involves the mitral valve or is located proximally, cardiac size is normal and there is right ventricular hypertrophy; if it occurs beyond the mitral valve, cardiomegaly is present, since there is usually left ventricular failure.

Regardless of the anatomic condition or the site of obstruction, certain predictable hemodynamic and related radiographic findings result. Increased pulmonary venous pressure causes enlarged upper-lobe pulmonary veins (cephalization). Increased pulmonary capillary pressure leads to pulmonary edema, with Kerley B lines. Increased pulmonary arterial pressure produces a dilated main pulmonary artery, and increased right ventricular pressure leads to right ventricular hypertrophy.

NORMAL HEART SIZE WITH NORMAL OR CONGESTIVE PULMONARY VASCULATURE

In this group of anomalies obstruction occurs at or proximal to the mitral valve. Left atrial enlargement may be present. The electrocardiogram shows isolated right ventricular hypertrophy.

Mitral Stenosis

Congenital mitral stenosis can be caused by either hypoplasia of the valve, as in the hypoplastic left heart syndrome, or a parachute mitral valve in which the chordae tendineae from both the valve leaflets converge into a single bulky papillary muscle. Radiographically, cardiac size is normal. Left atrial enlargement is present and, depending on the degree of mitral stenosis, right ventricular enlargement may be found. The main pulmonary artery segment is enlarged and the pulmonary vasculature can be normal or show venous congestion.

Supravalvular Ring of the Left Atrium

In this conditon, a fibrous ring encircles the left atrium immediately above the mitral valve. The left atrial appendage is located above the membrane. Hemodynamically and radiographically, this condition is identical to mitral stenosis. Supravalvular ring of the left atrium frequently coexists with a parachute mitral valve, coarctation of the aorta, or subvalvular aortic stenosis (Shone's syndrome).

Cor Triatriatum

In cor triatriatum there is an extra cardiac compartment that receives the pulmonary veins and is separated from the left atrium by a membrane with a central perforation. The left atrial appendage is located below the membrane. Embryologically, this condition represents incomplete incorporation of the pulmonary venous confluence into the left atrium. Hemodynamically and radiographically, the symptoms and signs resemble those of congenital mitral stenosis, but left atrial enlargement is often absent radiographically.

Stenosis of the Individual Pulmonary Veins

Atresia or hypoplasia of the pulmonary veins may occur at their junction with the left atrium. Hemodynamically, the signs resemble those of congenital mitral stenosis but are more severe. Radiographically, there is a pattern of severe passive congestion causing a reticular appearance throughout both lung fields. Left atrial enlargement is absent (Fig. 8–1).

Management. The membrane in cor triatriatum and in supravalvular stenosing ring may be resected. Among patients with mitral stenosis, it may be possible to perform a commissurotomy, but more commonly, because of the anatomic details, valve replacement is necessary. Catheter balloon dilatation may be effective in patients with stenosis of individual pulmonary veins.

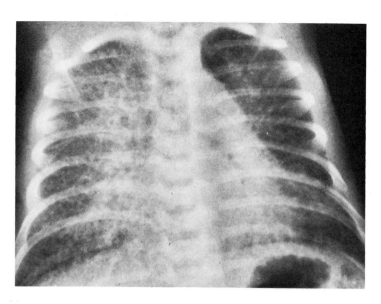

FIGURE 9–1. Neonate with stenosis of individual pulmonary veins. Coarse reticular pattern in both lung fields, more prominent in the right lung. Obliteration of right cardiac margin.

Selected Bibliography

Cor Triatriatum

Jacobstein, M. D., and Hirschfeld, S. S.: Concealed left atrial membrane: Pitfalls in the diagnosis of cor triatriatum and supravalve mitral ring. Am. J. Cardiol., *49*:780–786, 1982.

Marin-Garcia, J., Tandon, R., Lucas, R. V., and Edwards, J. E.: Cor triatriatum: Study of 20 cases. Am. J. Cardiol., *35*:59–66, 1975.

Atresia of the Pulmonary Vein

Levine, M. A., Moller, J. H., Amplatz, K., and Edwards, J. E.: Atresia of the common pulmonary vein: Case report and differential diagnosis. Am. J. Roentgenol., *2*:322–327, 1967.

CARDIOMEGALY WITH INCREASED PULMONARY VENOUS VASCULARITY

Cardiac conditions associated with left ventricular failure lead to a pattern of cardiomegaly, increased pulmonary venous vascularity, and left ventricular hypertrophy in the electrocardiogram. This combination can be caused either by a cardiomyopathy or by a left-sided obstructive lesion, such as severe aortic stenosis or coarctation of the aorta, which causes left ventricular failure.

Hypoplastic Left Heart Syndrome

The lesions caused by the underdevelopment of the left side of the heart include severe stenosis or atresia of the aortic or mitral valve, or both, and are

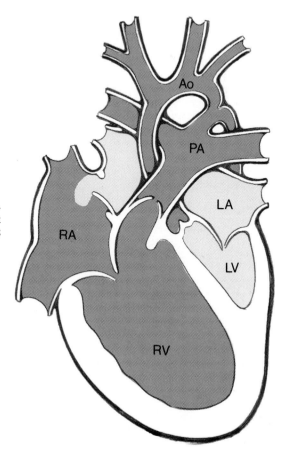

FIGURE 9–2. The central circulation, in aortic valvular atresia. Ao, Aorta; LA, left atrium; LV, left ventricle; PA, pulmonary artery; RA, right atrium; RV, right ventricle.

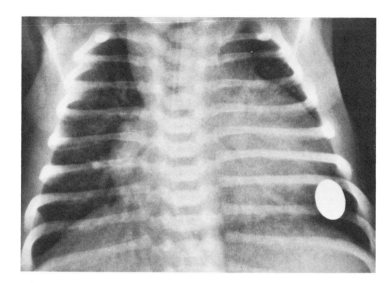

FIGURE 9–3. Coexistent aortic and mitral atresia. Increased pulmonary arterial vascularity. Congestive pattern. Haziness of the vascular markings. Cardiomegaly. Prominent right cardiac border.

associated with marked underdevelopment of the left atrium, left ventricle, and ascending aorta.

Hemodynamics (Fig. 9–2). Owing to the severe obstruction on the left side of the heart there is marked pulmonary venous hypertension, and consequently an obligatory left-to-right shunt either through a coexisting atrial septal defect or through a herniated foramen ovale. The blood reaches the right atrium through either one of these passages and passes through the right ventricle and out the pulmonary artery. Through a patent ductus arteriosus, the blood will then reach the systemic circulation.

Radiographic Features. The findings are variable, and in the first few hours of life some of the infants can show a normal cardiac size with pulmonary vascularity (Fig. 9–3). Within the first hour or so, or by the end of the first or second day, however, cardiomegaly and pulmonary vascular congestion become evident (Fig. 9–4).

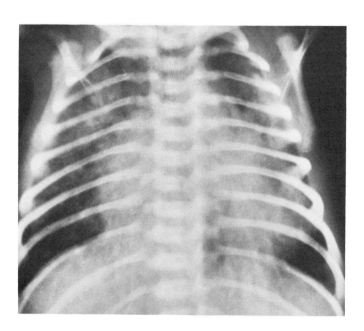

FIGURE 9–4. Aortic atresia. Pulmonary edema. Cardiomegaly. Prominent right cardiac border. Laterally displaced cardiac apex.

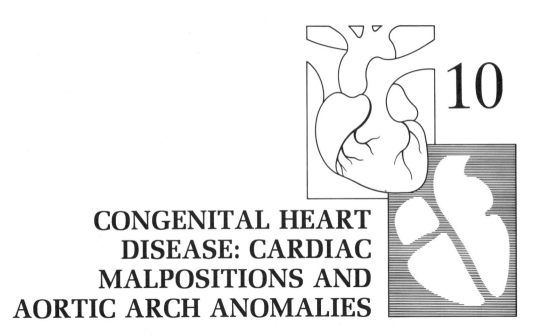

CONGENITAL HEART DISEASE: CARDIAC MALPOSITIONS AND AORTIC ARCH ANOMALIES

CARDIAC MALPOSITIONS

The heart may be abnormally located on either the right or the left side of the chest. The specific conditions are often initially recognized in a thoracic roentgenogram, and definite diagnosis of the cardiac malposition can usually be made accurately by analysis of the posteroanterior film.

In most individuals, certain basic anatomic relations exist. The inferior vena cava, major lobe of the liver, anatomic right atrium, and short stem bronchus are all present on the same side of the body; the descending aorta, anatomic left atrium, and stomach are present on the opposite side (Fig. 10–1). Usually, in a thoracic roentgenogram, some of these structures can be identified so that the patient's basic anatomic relations can be determined. In patients with situs solitus (the normal anatomic relations), the inferior vena cava, right atrium, short stem bronchus, and major hepatic lobe are on the patient's right side, while the cardiac apex, left atrium, descending aorta, and stomach are on the left side (Fig. 10–2). In patients with situs inversus, the opposite anatomic relations are present.

Rarely, these anatomic relations are not maintained. This state is considered discordant and is given the name "situs ambiguus" or "situs solitus indeterminus." Virtually all patients with situs ambiguus have either the asplenia or polysplenia syndrome.

Dextrocardia

Dextrocardia is a general term denoting the fact that the cardiac apex is located in the right hemithorax. There are five basic types.

1. Situs inversus heart, also called "mirror-image" dextrocardia. In this form, the basic anatomic features are those of situs inversus: the inferior vena cava, anatomic right atrium, and major lobe of the liver are on the left side and the

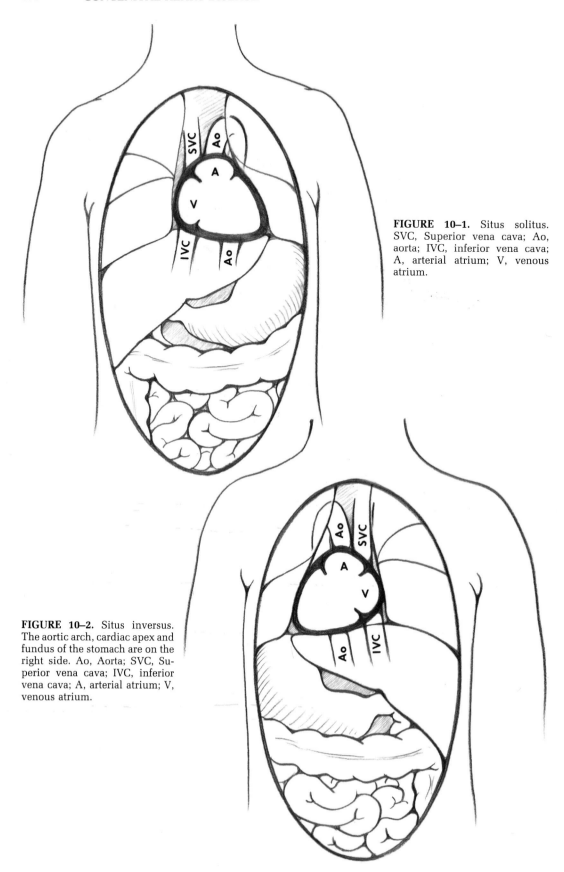

FIGURE 10–1. Situs solitus. SVC, Superior vena cava; Ao, aorta; IVC, inferior vena cava; A, arterial atrium; V, venous atrium.

FIGURE 10–2. Situs inversus. The aortic arch, cardiac apex and fundus of the stomach are on the right side. Ao, Aorta; SVC, Superior vena cava; IVC, inferior vena cava; A, arterial atrium; V, venous atrium.

cardiac apex, descending aorta, anatomic left atrium, and stomach are on the right side (Fig. 10–2). All visceral organs are positioned the opposite of normal. Thus there are three lobes in the left-sided lung and two lobes in the right-sided lung. The incidence of cardiac anomalies in patients with situs inversus is greater than in patients with situs solitus, being present in 5 to 10 per cent. These anomalies are often complicated and include conditions such as transposition of great vessels or single ventricle.

Kartagener's syndrome is a combination of situs inversus, bronchiectasis, and sinusitis. Abnormalities of the cilia are also present, which can explain the respiratory complications, but the relation of this finding to the abnormal situs remains unclear.

The electrocardiogram is typical in that the limb leads appear the opposite of normal. The thoracic roentgenogram also shows the reverse of normal; the aortic arch, cardiac apex, and stomach bubble are located on the right side.

2. Dextroposition of situs solitus. In this condition, the basic anatomic relations are those of situs solitus, but the heart is displaced into the right hemithorax because of an extrinsic factor, usually either hypoplasia or agenesis of the right lung. The degree of displacement is variable and depends on the reduction in the volume of the right lung (Fig. 10–3).

Many patients have coexistent cardiac conditions, particularly those associated with left-to-right shunts. These patients have a tendency to pulmonary hyperten-

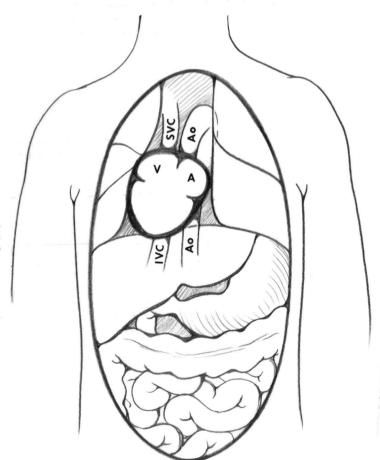

FIGURE 10–3. Dextroposition. Ao, Aorta; SVC, superior vena cava; IVC, inferior vena cava; A, arterial atrium; V, venous atrium.

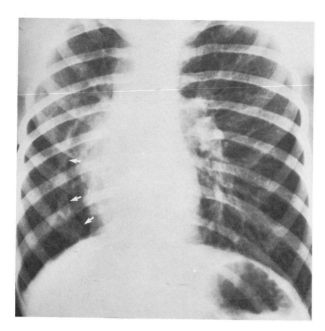

FIGURE 10–4. Scimitar syndrome. Thoracic roentgenogram. Posteroanterior projection. Asymmetry of the thorax. Right hemithorax smaller than left. Mediastinum shifted toward right. Cardiac apex on left. Vascular shadow in right lower lung field joins inferior vena cava (white arrows).

venolobar syndrome

sion, probably because of the reduced cross-sectional area of the pulmonary arterial tree. One unusual syndrome associated with dextroposition, the scimitar syndrome. also includes hypoplasia of the right lung, partial anomalous pulmonary venous connection to the inferior vena cava, and arteries arising from the descending aorta passing to the right lower lobe. Intracardiac anomalies are common. The syndrome derives its name from the characteristic curvilinear density in the right lung, representing the anomalous venous connection of the lung with the inferior vena cava, which has the shape of the famous Turkish sword (Fig. 10–4). The diagnosis is made by cardiac catheterization and angiography.

3. Dextroversion of situs solitus. In this condition, the basic anatomic relations are normal (situs solitus), but the cardiac apex is in the right side of the chest (Fig. 10–5). The dextroversion results from an abnormality in the rotation of the embryonic cardiac loop. In some patients, a D-ventricular loop is present and the primitive bulboventricular loop remains in the right hemithorax. Most of these patients have complex congenital cardiac anomalies. In the others, an L-ventricular loop is present, a result of the primitive bulboventricular loop having initially rotated toward the left and then migrated into the right hemithorax. These patients have corrected transposition of the great vessels and its associated anomalies.

The radiographic diagnosis is made on the basis of the presence of the cardiac apex in the right hemithorax, while the aortic arch and stomach bubble are on the left side (Fig. 10–6).

4. Dextrocardia with situs ambiguus secondary to asplenia syndrome (Fig. 10–7). The asplenia syndrome has also been called bilateral rightsidedness because of the anatomic form of the visceral anomalies. The spleen, normally a left-sided organ, is absent; both lungs have three lobes; and the left lobe of the liver is the same size as the right lobe (Fig. 10–8). Interestingly, most patients have malrotation of the bowel, with either nonrotation or reverse rotation of the mid-gut loop.

Cardiac anomalies, usually complex and multiple, are almost always present. The most common anomalies are single atrium, single ventricle, pulmonary stenosis or atresia, transposition of the great vessels, total anomalous pulmonary

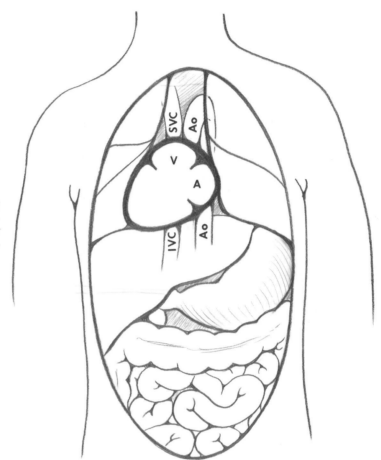

FIGURE 10–5. Dextroversion of situs solitus. Ao, Aorta; SVC, superior vena cava; IVC, inferior vena cava; A, arterial atrium; V, venous atrium.

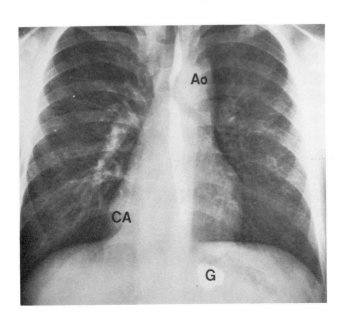

FIGURE 10–6. Dextroversion of situs solitus. Aortic arch (Ao) and gastric fundus (G) on left side. Cardiac apex (CA) on right side.

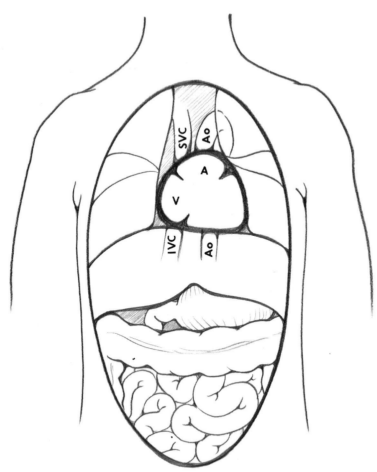

FIGURE 10–7. Asplenia. Ao, Aorta; SVC, superior vena cava; IVC, inferior vena cava; A, arterial atrium; V, venous atrium.

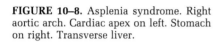

FIGURE 10–8. Asplenia syndrome. Right aortic arch. Cardiac apex on left. Stomach on right. Transverse liver.

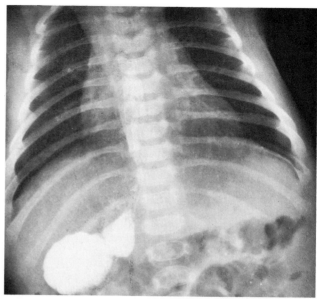

venous connection, and bilateral superior venae cavae. In one half of the patients, the heart is in the right hemithorax.

The radiograph typically shows a horizontal lower hepatic margin, and the liver occupies the entire upper abdomen (Fig. 10–8). Minor lobe fissures may be seen in each lung. The cardiac apex may be located in either hemithorax. Usually, cardiac size is normal and pulmonary vascularity decreased. If catheters are present in both the aorta and inferior vena cava, they lie on the same side rather than on opposite sides of the spine.

5. Dextrocardia with situs ambiguus secondary to the polysplenia syndrome. The polysplenia syndrome has also been called bilateral leftsidedness; each lung has two lobes and hyparterial bronchi, the spleen consists of multiple masses, and the hepatic segment of the inferior vena cava is absent (Fig. 10–9). Malrotation of the bowel is also found. Cardiac anomalies are likewise common but are usually less complex than in asplenia. The anomalies include atrial septal defect, occasionally of the ostium primum type; partial anomalous pulmonary venous connection; interrupted inferior vena cava with azygous continuation; bilateral superior venae cavae; and a left-sided outflow lesion. In about one half of the cases, the heart is in the right hemithorax. Since each lung has only two lobes, minor pulmonary tissue is not observed.

This condition should be suspected in patients with an unusual pattern of malposition and increased pulmonary vasculature, particularly if there is an enlarged azygos vein.

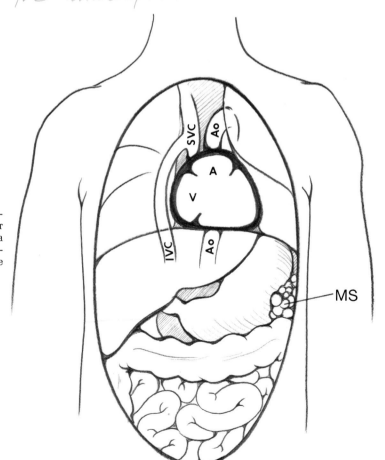

FIGURE 10–9. Polysplenia syndrome. Ao, Aorta; SVC, superior vena cava; IVC, inferior vena cava; A, arterial atrium; V, venous atrium; MS, multiple spleens.

Levocardia

The heart may also be malpositioned in the left hemithorax. Five conditions are associated with levocardia.

1. Situs solitus. This is the normal anatomic arrangement.

2. Levoversion of situs inversus (Fig. 10–10). This rare condition is the opposite of dextroversion of situs solitus. Corrected transposition of the great vessels is almost always present. Radiographically, levoversion of situs inversus is recognized because the heart is in the left hemithorax, but the abdominal contents show situs inversus (Fig. 10–11).

3. Levoposition of situs solitus (Fig. 10–12). In this situation the organs show situs solitus, but the heart is displaced further into the left chest because of hypoplasia of the left lung. As in dextroposition, pulmonary hypertension may occur if there is a left-to-right shunt. The condition can be suspected radiographically because the left hemithorax is smaller than the right and the left intercostal spaces are narrower (Fig. 10–13).

4. Levocardia with situs ambiguus secondary to asplenia syndrome. This is recognized radiographically by means of the asplenia.

5. Levocardia with situs ambiguus secondary to polysplenia syndrome. This is recognized radiographically by means of the polysplenia.

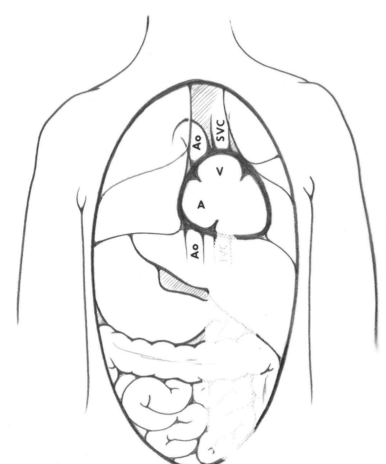

FIGURE 10–10. Levoversion of situs inversus. Ao, Aorta; SVC, superior vena cava; IVC, inferior vena cava; A, arterial atrium; V, venous atrium.

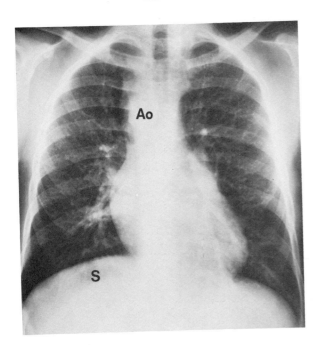

FIGURE 10–11. Levoversion of situs inversus. Aortic arch (Ao) on right, indenting trachea toward left. Stomach fundus on right (S). Cardiac apex on left. Normal pulmonary vascularity. Normal cardiac size.

FIGURE 10–12. Levoposition of situs solitus. Ao, Aorta; SVC, superior vena cava; IVC, inferior vena cava; A, arterial atrium; V, venous atrium.

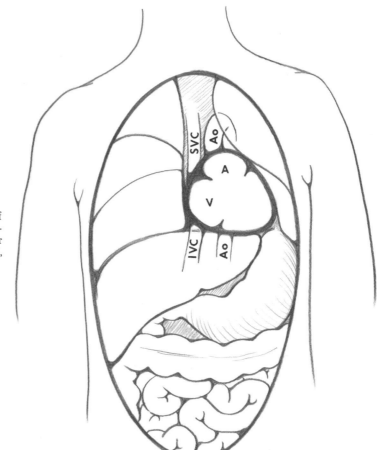

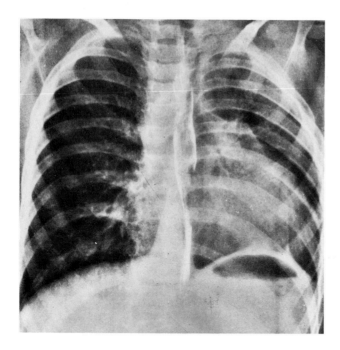

FIGURE 10–13. Interruption of left pulmonary artery. Levoposition of heart. Asymmetrical thorax. Decreased width of intercostal spaces and decreased size of left hemithorax. Mediastinum shifted to the left. Asymmetry of vascular markings, more prominent in the right lung field. Right aortic arch. Gastric fundus on the right.

Selected Bibliography

Anselmi, G., Munoz, S., Blanco, P., Machado, I., and de la Cruz, M. V.: Systematization and clinical study of dextroversion, mirror-image dextrocardia, and laevoversion. Br. Heart J., 34:1085–1098, 1972.

Arcilla, R. A., and Gasul, B. M.: Congenital dextrocardia: Clinical, angiocardiographic, and autopsy studies on 50 patients. J. Pediatr., 58(1):39–58, 1961, and 58(2):251–262, 1961.

Carey, L. S., and Edwards, J. E.: Roentgenographic, angiocardiographic and pathologic findings in congenital cardiac disease associated with agenesis of the spleen. Am. J. Roentgenol., 91(4):885–890, 1964.

Farnsworth, A. E., and Ankeney, J. L.: The spectrum of the scimitar syndrome. J. Thorac. Cardiovasc. Surg., 68:37–42, 1974.

Felson, B.: The many faces of pulmonary sequestration. Semin. Roentgenol., 7:3–16, 1972.

Kiely, B., Filler, J., Stone, S., and Doyle, E. F.: Syndromes of anomalous venous drainage of the right lung to the inferior vena cava. A review of 67 reported cases and three new cases in children. Am. J. Cardiol., 20:102–116, 1967.

Rao, P. S.: Dextrocardia: Systematic approach to differential diagnosis. Am. Heart J., 102:389–403, 1981.

Rohem, J. O. F., June, K. L., and Amplatz, K.: Radiographic features of the scimitar syndrome. Radiology, 86:856–859, 1966.

Ruttenberg, H. D., Neufeld, H. N., Lucas, R. V., Jr., Carey, L. S., Adams, P., Anderson, R. C., and Edwards, J. E.: Syndrome of congenital cardiac disease with asplenia: Distinction from other forms of congenital cyanotic cardiac disease. Am. J. Cardiol., 13(3):387–406, 1964.

Squarcia, U., Ritter, D. G., and Kincaid, O. W.: Dextrocardia: Angiocardiographic study and classification. Am. J. Cardiol., 32:965–977, 1973.

Wagenvoort, C. A., Heath, D., and Edwards, J. E.: The pathology of the pulmonary vasculature. Springfield, IL, Charles C Thomas, 1964, p. 392.

AORTIC ARCH ANOMALIES

Several anomalies in the formation of the aortic arch can be identified either on the thoracic roentgenogram or by means of a barium swallow; thus, identification of the aortic arch is a necessary part of the interpretation of any thoracic roentgenogram.

Embryology. Early in embryologic development, the first major arterial vessels, the paired dorsal aortae, lie on either side of the foregut (see Fig. 1–9). Because of the relative change of the position of the cardiogenic plate, the proximal portions of these dorsal aortae form arches. The dorsal aortae join the primitive common truncus in a structure called the aortic sac. The arches formed by the dorsal aortae represent the paired first aortic arches. From the aortic sac, five other paired arches subsequently develop, but not all are present simultaneously.

Although remnants of the first, second, and third paired arches persist at birth, the fourth and sixth arches form major cardiovascular structures, namely the aortic arch and the proximal pulmonary arteries, respectively. Serious anomalies may occur in the formation of these two arches.

Abnormalities of the Fourth Aortic Arches

Almost all abnormalities of the aortic arch system can be explained by the hypothetical double aortic arch proposed by Edwards. Early in development, there are paired fourth aortic arches, which arise from the ascending aorta, pass on either side of the trachea and esophagus, and join to enter one of the dorsal aortae. From each arch, the ipsilateral common carotid and subclavian arteries arise. Usually, the right dorsal aorta regresses and the left dorsal aorta persists. The various anomalies result either from failure of regression or from abnormal site of regression of the aortic arch.

Double Aortic Arch

Double aortic arch results from failure in regression in either arch. As a result, the trachea and esophagus are encircled by the aortic arches, and symptoms

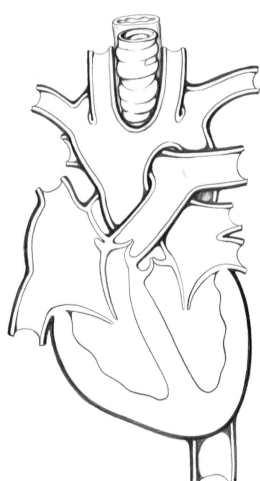

FIGURE 10–14. Double aortic arch.

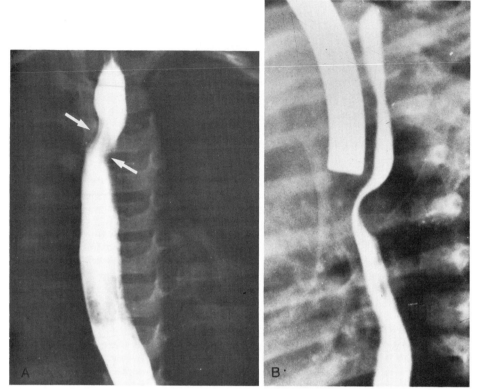

FIGURE 10–15. Double aortic arch. *A,* Thoracic roentgenogram. Posteroanterior projection. Barium swallow shows indentations of both walls of esophagus, right larger than left. *B,* Marked posterior indentation on esophagus. Tracheostomy cannula present because of severe tracheal obstruction.

result from their compression (Fig. 10–14). Usually, the descending aorta descends in the left hemithorax. The right aortic arch, which is usually larger, passes posterior to the esophagus, while the smaller left aortic arch is located anterior to the trachea. Occasionally, the anterior arch is atretic and represented by a fibrous band. The brachiocephalic arteries are arranged symmetrically; the common carotid arteries arise anteriorly and the subcalvian arteries arise posteriorly from the respective aortic arches. The ductus arteriosus may connect to either subclavian artery. Double aortic arch usually occurs as an isolated anomaly without congenital cardiac malformation.

Radiographic Features. In the posteroanterior projection, the trachea is not displaced and is located in the midline, since it is fixed laterally by the two arches and therefore cannot deviate. In a lateral projection, the trachea is displaced posteriorly and narrowed. In a posteroanterior projection, the esophagus is indented on both sides, with the indentation caused by the right arch being located slightly higher than that caused by the left arch (Fig. 10–15*A*). The esophagus is also indented posteriorly as the right arch crosses obliquely to join the left arch (Fig. 10–15*B*).

Angiographic Appearance. Aortography in the long-axial oblique projection will show the double arch better than in an anteroposterior projection (Fig. 10–16).

Management. Since most patients with this anomaly have dysphagia and stridor, the smaller arch (usually the anterior one) is divided, thereby decompressing the ring.

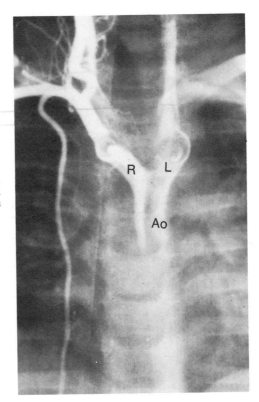

FIGURE 10–16. Double aortic arch. Retrograde aortogram. Origin of right subclavian and right carotid arteries from right arch (R) and left subclavian and left carotid arteries from left arch (L). Ascending aorta (Ao).

Left Aortic Arch

Left aortic arch results from regression in the right aortic arch and is formed by persistence of both the left aortic arch and the left dorsal aorta. A left aortic arch passes to the left of the trachea and esophagus and above the left mainstem bronchus.

Radiographic Features. A left aortic arch can be recognized by observing the rightward displacement of the tracheal air column by the aortic arch. Since the aortic arch crosses obliquely from an anterior to a posterior position, the trachea is displaced more to the right than the esophagus and thus lies to the right of the barium-filled esophagus (see Fig. 4–2).

Depending on the site of regression in the right aortic arch, two variations of left aortic arch result and are described according to the presence or absence of a retroesophageal vessel.

1. Without retroesophageal segment (Fig. 10–17). This represents a normal aortic arch. In embryo, regression occurs in the right aortic arch beyond the right subclavian artery. The first brachiocephalic vessel arising from the left aortic arch is the innominate artery, giving rise to the right subclavian and right carotid arteries. The arch next gives oxygen successively to the left carotid and the left subclavian arteries. There is no aortic arch remnant behind the esophagus. On a lateral view of a barium swallow, therefore, the esophagus is not displaced.

2. With retroesophageal segment (left aortic arch with aberrant right subclavian artery) (Fig. 10–18). This anomaly results from regression of the right fourth aortic arch between the right carotid and right subclavian arteries; thus the right subclavian artery arises from the proximal descending aorta and passes behind

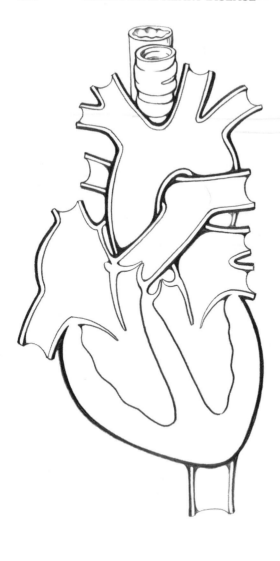

FIGURE 10–17. Normal aortic arch.

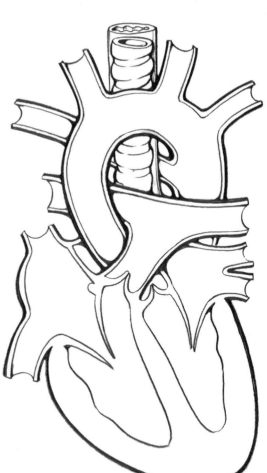

FIGURE 10–18. Left aortic arch and aberrant right subclavian artery.

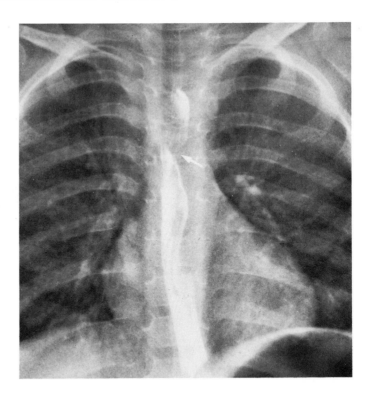

FIGURE 10–19. Aortic arch with aberrant right subclavian artery, indenting the barium column obliquely upward (arrow).

the esophagus obliquely and superiorly toward the right arm. These patients are asymptomatic, since the trachea and esophagus are not encircled by vascular structures. The aberrant right subclavian artery is evident in a posteroanterior roentgenogram as a radiolucent band crossing the esophagus obliquely upward toward the right shoulder. In a lateral or left anterior oblique projection, a shallow, posterior indentation is present in the barium-filled esophagus (Fig. 10–19).

Right Aortic Arch

Right aortic arch results from regression in the left aortic arch and is formed by persistence of the right arch and right descending aorta. The arch passes to the right of the trachea and esophagus and over the right mainstem bronchus (Fig. 10–20). It descends in the right thorax but usually crosses the lower thoracic spine to pass through the left hemidiaphragm.

Radiographically, the barium-filled esophagus is located to the right of the trachea and the trachea may be deviated slightly to the left. The proximal descending aorta may be seen on the right of the spine.

Two varieties of right aortic arch occur, depending on the site of regression.

1. Without retroesophageal segment (Fig. 10–20). This is a mirror image of a left aortic arch and results from regression of the distal left aortic arch beyond the left subclavian artery. Right aortic arch without a retroesophageal segment is almost always associated with congenital heart disease, most commonly tetralogy of Fallot; persistent truncus arteriosus; or ventricular septal defect with infundibular pulmonary stenosis.

2. With retroesophageal segment (right arch with an aberrant left subclavian

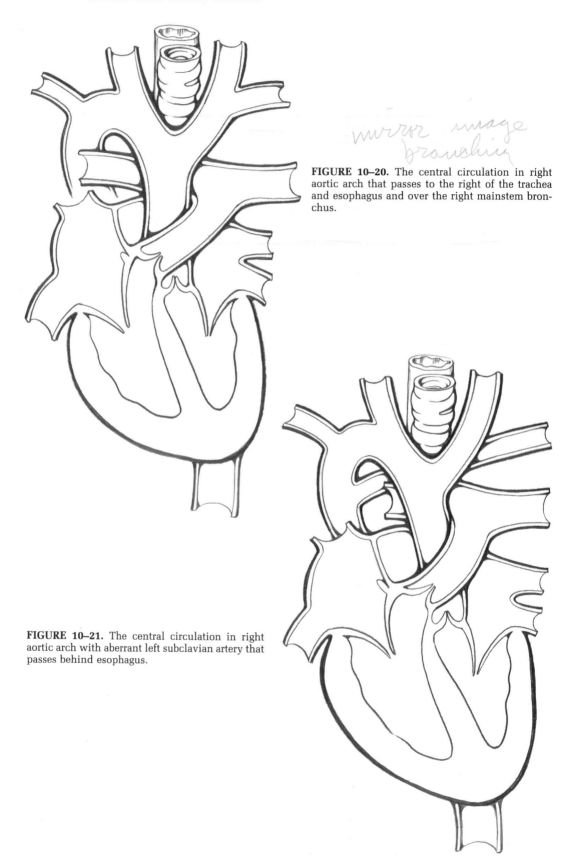

mirror image branching

FIGURE 10–20. The central circulation in right aortic arch that passes to the right of the trachea and esophagus and over the right mainstem bronchus.

FIGURE 10–21. The central circulation in right aortic arch with aberrant left subclavian artery that passes behind esophagus.

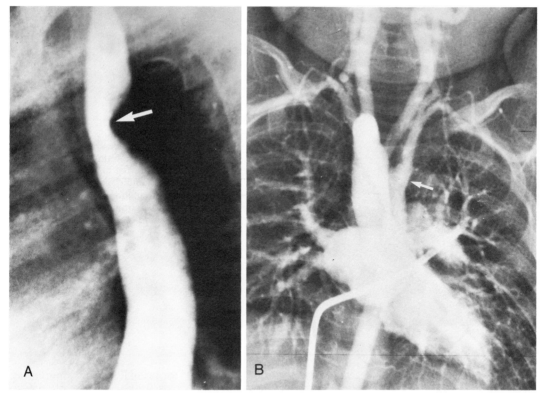

FIGURE 10–22. Right aortic arch with aberrant left subclavian artery. *A,* Wide posterior indentation of barium column (arrow). *B,* Pulmonary arteriogram in anteroposterior projection. Right aortic arch. Aorta crosses to left, causing posterior indentation of barium column. Aberrant left subclavian artery arises from large aortic diverticulum (arrow).

artery) (Fig. 10–21). This condition results from regression of the left fourth aortic arch between the left common carotid and left subclavian arteries. The aberrant left subclavian artery arises from an aortic diverticulum of the proximal descending aorta and passes obliquely and superiorly to the left arm (Fig. 10–22). In a barium swallow, the diverticulum causes a broad indentation on the posterior wall of the esophagus or, on a posteroanterior view, a radiolucency that is directed obliquely and superiorly toward the left arm. In patients with tetralogy of Fallot, the aberrant left subclavian artery does not arise from an aortic diverticulum because ductal flow was small in utero. If a ductus arteriosus arises from the aberrant left subclavian artery, a vascular ring results. The combination of right aortic arch, aberrant left subclavian artery, and left ductus arteriosus is the most common type of right arch and is usually unassociated with congenital heart disease.

In some patients with right aortic arch with aberrant left subclavian artery, a vascular ring is completed by a left-sided ductus arteriosus, either ligamentous or patent. Division of the ductus alleviates the symptoms of the vascular ring.

Abnormalities of the Sixth Aortic Arch

Abnormalities of the sixth aortic arch are much less common, the most important being pulmonary artery sling. This anomaly, also called origin of the left pulmonary artery from the right pulmonary artery, results from a failure of

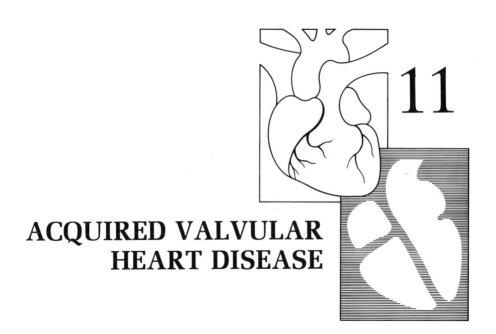

ACQUIRED VALVULAR
HEART DISEASE

The cardiac valves may be damaged by various diseases that lead to either stenosis or insufficiency. The aortic and mitral valves are most commonly affected; the underlying cause may be congenital or acquired. Tricuspid valvular disease occurs occasionally; pulmonary valvular abnormality, other than congenital, is rare.

Regardless of the valve involved, the principal hemodynamic effect of valvular stenosis is an increase in the pressure in the proximal cardiac chamber during the period of the cardiac cycle when the valve is open. Thus, in aortic stenosis, the left ventricular pressure is elevated during systole; in mitral stenosis, the left atrial pressure is increased during diastole. The heart responds to an increase in pressure by hypertrophy, *not* dilatation. Usually, cardiac size is normal until decompensation occurs; then cardiomegaly develops.

Valvular insufficiency causes enlargement of the cardiac chambers on both sides of the insufficient valve regardless of the valve involved. The primary cardiac response to an insufficient valve is dilatation, and cardiac enlargement is therefore present on the roentgenogram.

MITRAL VALVE DISEASE

Rheumatic fever is the primary cause of symptomatic mitral valvular disease. During acute rheumatic fever, the inflammatory process may involve the heart. Later, over a period of years, chronic thickening and fibrosis of the mitral valve leaflets, and fusion and shortening of the chordae tendineae, occur. Mitral valve damage due to rheumatic fever is much more prevalent in females than in males.

Stenosis

Mitral stenosis is almost always the result of rheumatic fever. It is the product of fusion of the valve leaflets at their commissures, and fusion and shortening of the chordae tendineae. Rare causes of mitral stenosis are bacterial endocarditis, with obstruction of the orifice by large vegetations; atrial thrombi or tumors obstructing the mitral valvular orifice; and congenital anomalies.

195

Hemodynamics. In an adult the mitral valve normally has an area of 4 to 6 sq cm. The normal orifice can accommodate a greatly increased flow, as occurs during exercise, without an increase in the left atrial pressure, which is normally 10 mm Hg. When the area of the orifice is reduced to 1.5 sq cm, there is a slight increase in the left atrial pressure that is accentuated during exercise. When the orifice is 0.5 sq cm, left atrial pressure at rest is 35 mm Hg and minimal exertion causes a marked increase.

Thus, in mitral stenosis the left atrium is hypertrophied and enlarged. The elevated left atrial pressure and the consequent left atrial–left ventricular gradient, particularly during late diastole when the atrium contracts, discharge blood into the left ventricle. Because of the elevated left atrial pressure, the pulmonary capillary pressure is increased; when it reaches 30 to 35 mm Hg, pulmonary edema develops.

Pulmonary arterial pressure is elevated. In many patients, this increase is proportional to the elevated left atrial pressure; in patients with more severe stenosis the elevation is disproportionate because of pulmonary arteriolar hypertrophy. This marked increase in pulmonary arterial pressure causes right ventricular hypertrophy and occasionally right ventricular failure. The marked elevation of pulmonary arteriolar resistance is advantageous, however, since it limits the pulmonary blood flow and protects the lungs from abrupt increases in pulmonary capillary pressure and pulmonary edema.

Clinical Features. The principal symptom of mitral stenosis is dyspnea, which initially occurs only on exertion, but later is also present when the patient rests or reclines. Episodes of pulmonary edema may occur. Palpitations may occur when atrial fibrillation occurs, secondary to left atrial enlargement. Symptoms of either systemic or pulmonary embolism may occur in patients with atrial fibrillation.

The cardinal auscultatory findings are a loud first heart sound (mitral closure), an open snap, a mid-diastolic murmur, and a crescendo late diastolic murmur. The pulmonary component of the second heart sound is loud if pulmonary hypertension is present. The cardiac rhythm may be irregular because of atrial fibrillation. The electrocardiogram shows the broad notched P waves of left atrial enlargement, as well as right ventricular hypertrophy. Atrial fibrillation is common.

Echocardiographic Features. The left atrial dimension is increased, whereas that of the left ventricle is normal or decreased. Right ventricular hypertrophy and enlargement are present in patients with pulmonary hypertension.

Multiple echoes may be recorded from the mitral valve, and the EF slope characteristically is low (Fig. 11–1). The posterior mitral valve leaflet moves anteriorly during diastole. On cross-sectional echocardiography, the movement of

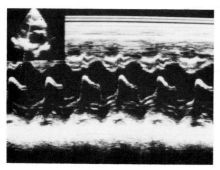

IVS

LV

LVPW

FIGURE 11–1. Mitral stenosis. M-mode echocardiogram with projection through interventricular septum (IVS), left ventricle (LV), and left ventricular posterior wall (LVPW). Low E to F slope during diastole.

the mitral valve leaflets is restricted, and they do not move fully toward the walls of the left ventricle during diastole.

Radiographic Features. The radiographic appearance of the heart and lungs in mitral stenosis varies with the severity of the stenosis. In mild mitral stenosis, cardiac size and contour and the pulmonary vasculature are all normal (Fig. 11–2).

In moderate mitral stenosis the cardiac size is normal. Left atrial enlargement, however, is present and causes (1) a bulge representing the left atrial appendage located below the pulmonary artery or the left cardiac border and (2) posterior displacement of the barium-filled esophagus. In the left anterior oblique projection, left atrial enlargement causes fullness below the left mainstem bronchus. The left ventricle is small. Slight signs of pulmonary venous obstruction are present (Fig. 11–3).

In severe mitral stenosis the heart is enlarged, partly as a result of right atrial enlargement and right ventricular failure. There are signs of pulmonary venous obstruction and other changes in the pulmonary vascular bed. The left mainstem bronchus is elevated by the enlarged left atrium, a feature that is seen best on a left anterior oblique projection (Fig. 11–3).

The obstruction at the mitral valve level, depending on its severity and duration, causes changes in the pulmonary vascular bed that may be subdivided into three categories. First, there are signs of pulmonary venous hypertension (Fig. 11–3): (1) narrowing of vascular markings in the lower lung fields and (2) prominent vascular markings in the upper lung fields caused by distention of the pulmonary veins.

As the severity of the obstruction increases, there is further progression of the vascular changes, manifested by signs of pulmonary capillary hypertension (Figs. 11–4 and 11–5): (1) Kerley A and B lines in the lower lobes, (2) perivascular haziness because of pulmonary edema, and (3) loss of translucency in the lung bases due to pulmonary edema.

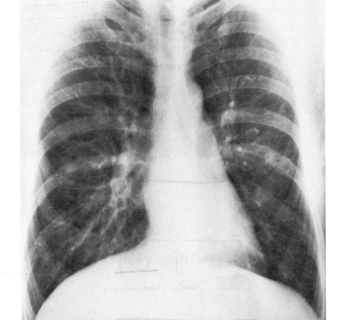

FIGURE 11–2. Mild mitral stenosis. Normal pulmonary vascularity. Normal cardiac size.

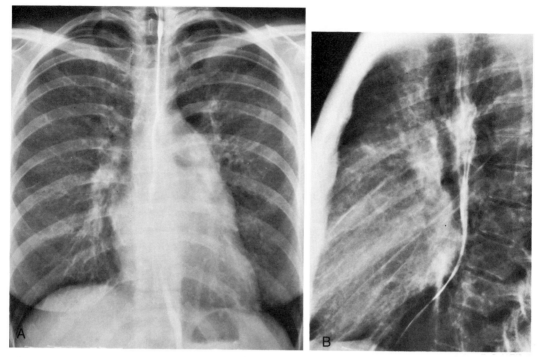

Figure 11–3. Moderate mitral stenosis. *A,* Posteroanterior projection. Prominent vascular markings in upper lobes are a manifestation of redistribution of blood flow toward the upper lobes. Normal cardiac size. Left atrial enlargement, manifested by double density, prominent left atrial appendage, and slight displacement of esophagus toward the right. Prominent main pulmonary artery segment. *B,* Lateral projection. Marked enlargement of left atrium. Displacement of the barium-filled esophagus posteriorly. Partial obliteration of retrosternal space by enlarged right ventricle.

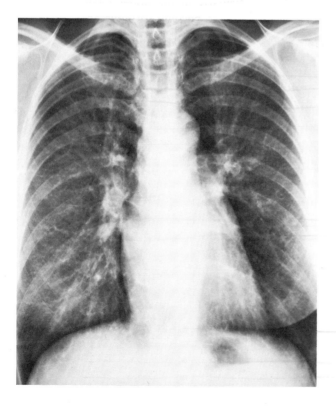

FIGURE 11–4. More severe mitral stenosis. Kerley B lines in both lung fields. Indistinctness of vascular markings and redistribution of blood flow toward the upper lobes. Large central hilar vessels. Normal cardiac size. Left atrial enlargement, indicated by double density in area of left atrium and prominent left atrial appendage.

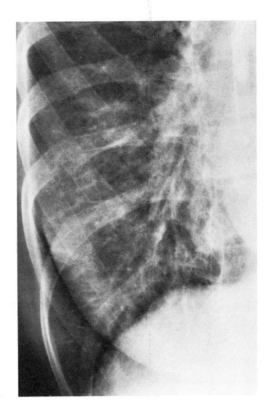

FIGURE 11–5. Mitral stenosis. Kerley B lines in right lung field.

Finally, when fixed pulmonary vascular changes supervene, signs of pulmonary arterial hypertension appears: (1) the main pulmonary artery segment becomes prominent; (2) the central pulmonary arteries, particularly in the upper lobes, become enlarged; and (3) the smaller pulmonary arteries become tortuous and have a rapid tapering of branches into the mid-lung areas.

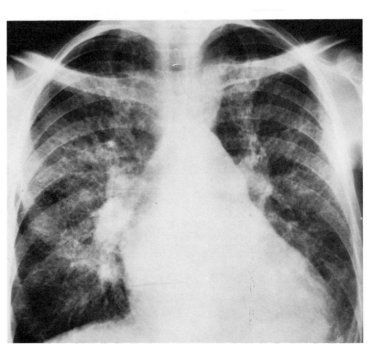

FIGURE 11–6. Long-standing mitral stenosis. Small bilateral pleural effusions. Kerley B lines and diffuse nodularity throughout both lung fields. Prominent vascular markings in upper lobes. Large hilar vessels. Cardiomegaly. Left atrial enlargement manifested as a double density. Prominent main pulmonary artery segment.

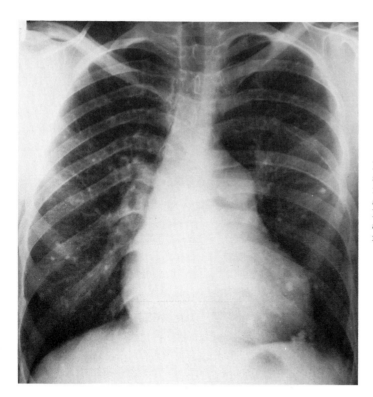

FIGURE 11–7. Long-standing mitral stenosis. Multiple calcified nodules in both lung fields, more abundant at the bases. Mild cardiomegaly. Flattening of segment of left atrial appendage. Prominent main pulmonary artery segment.

In long-standing mitral stenosis and pulmonary congestion, hemosiderin is deposited in the lungs, causing nodular densities or reticular areas resembling those of miliary tuberculosis or pneumonoconiosis (Fig. 11–6). These nodules may calcify or ossify, appearing as multiple, dense opacities scattered throughout the lung bases (Fig. 11–7).

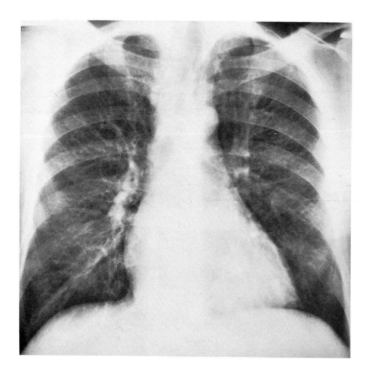

FIGURE 11–8. Mitral stenosis. Kerley B lines. Indistinct vascular markings in lower lobes and prominent vascular markings in upper lobes. Cardiac size at upper limit of normal.

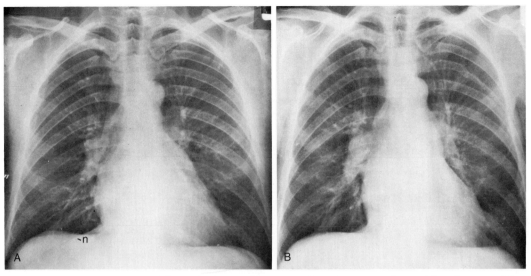

FIGURE 11–9. *A,* Before mitral commissurotomy. Prominent vascular markings in upper lobes. Mild cardiomegaly. Prominent left atrial appendage area. *B,* Following mitral commissurotomy. Prominent vascular markings in upper lobes. Large hilar vessels. Cardiac size is unchanged. Flattening of the left atrial appendage segment secondary to surgical procedure.

Acute obstruction of the mitral orifice by an atrial thrombus, an atrial tumor, or a large vegetation (in bacterial endocarditis) causes sudden elevation of the left atrial pressure and pulmonary edema. These signs may disappear as abruptly as they appeared when the valvular obstruction is relieved (Fig. 11–8).

Angiographic Features. Left ventriculography with a shallow right anterior oblique projection demonstrates a doming, thickened mitral valve.

Management. In patients with symptomatic mitral stenosis, the obstruction is relieved by mitral commissurotomy, if the leaflets are pliable (Fig. 11–9), or mitral valve replacement if not (Fig. 11–10).

Mitral Insufficiency

Rheumatic fever is the leading cause of symptomatic mitral insufficiency. The rheumatic process fuses and shortens the chordae tendineae, which limits the movements of the valvular leaflets and prevents complete closure of the orifice during systole. The condition is usually associated with some degree of mitral stenosis. Other causes of mitral insufficiency include rupture of papillary muscle as a result of myocardial infarction or bacterial endocarditis, perforation of a valve cusp or rupture of chordae tendineae as the result of bacterial endocarditis, and Marfan's syndrome. Mitral insufficiency may also occur secondary to disease causing left ventricular failure, such as systemic hypertension, coronary artery disease, and aortic valvular disease. Mitral insufficiency in this instance may result from either dilatation of the mitral valve ring or tethering of the cusps by the chordae tendineae, which are stretched taut as the left ventricle elongates.

The leading cause of mitral insufficiency is mitral valve prolapse, in which the posterior leaflet prolapses into the left atrium during mid to late diastole. This condition, which is reported to affect 7 per cent of females, usually permits only minimal regurgitation and rarely produces significant hemodynamic abnormalities.

Hemodynamics. The degree of mitral regurgitation depends on the extent of

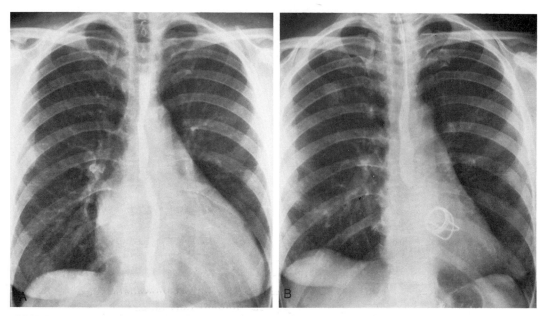

FIGURE 11–10. *A*, Before mitral valve replacement with Starr-Edwards prosthesis. Prominent vascular markings in upper lobes. Cardiomegaly. Left atrial enlargement evidenced by double density and displacement of the barium-filled esophagus toward the left. *B*, Following valve replacement. Normal pulmonary vascularity. Normal cardiac size. Starr-Edwards valve prosthesis in mitral position.

the mitral valve that is not occluded by tissue during systole, the pressure difference between the left ventricular and atrium during systole, and the impedence to left ventricular outflow. Even if the unguarded area in the mitral valve is small compared to the size of the aortic valve orifice, the volume of reflux may be large, because the left atrial pressure is considerably lower than the aortic pressure.

Because of mitral regurgitation, the volume of blood flow into the left atrium is increased. Therefore, the left atrium dilates and, in patients with severe mitral insufficiency, it may contain 2 to 3 liters of blood. During diastole there is an increased flow of blood from the left atrium into the left ventricle, the volume equaling the cardiac output plus the regurgitant volume. Therefore, the left ventricle dilates and has an increased diastolic volume. According to Starling's law, this increase in diastolic volume causes a more forceful contraction in order to maintain the cardiac output.

Mitral insufficiency is complicated by dilatation of both the left atrium and the left ventricle and secondary hypertrophy of these chambers. With progressive left ventricular dilatation, the amount of mitral regurgitation tends to increase, which further dilates the left ventricle. Eventually, the left ventricle decompensates.

Left atrial pressure increases because of the increased left atrial volume. The level of left atrial pressure depends on the compliance of the left atrial wall and the suddenness of the appearance of mitral insufficiency. Sudden mitral insufficiency causes a sharp increase in left atrial pressure because the left atrium is suddenly distended. In contrast, the more common progression of mitral regurgitation allows gradual dilatation of the left atrium and thus causes a smaller increase in left atrial pressure.

As left atrial pressure increases, pulmonary venous pressure also increases; subsequently, the pulmonary arterial and right ventricular systolic pressures rise.

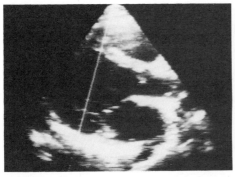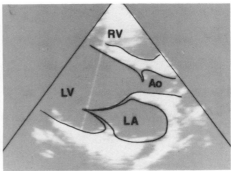

FIGURE 11–11. Mitral insufficiency. Cross-sectional echocardiogram. Long axis-view. Dilated left ventricle. RV, Right ventricle; LV, left ventricle; Ao, aorta; LA, left atrium.

Usually, the pressures attained are not so high as those in patients with mitral stenosis. Right ventricular failure rarely occurs.

Clinical Features. Patients with mitral insufficiency are asymptomatic for a long time but eventually have fatigue and dyspnea—initially only on exertion and then at rest. There is clinical evidence of cardiomegaly and increased cardiac activity. An apical pansystolic murmur of the murmur correlates with the degree of mitral regurgitation. A mid-diastolic murmur, present in many patients, is caused by increased antegrade flow across the mitral valve and does not signify coexistent stenosis. The pulmonary component of the second heart sound may be accentuated if pulmonary hypertension is present.

In patients with mitral valve prolapse, the murmur begins in mid to late systole and is initiated by a mid-systolic click.

Echocardiographic Features. The echocardiogram is not diagnostic of mitral regurgitation. On M-mode and cross-sectional echocardiograms, both the left atrium and left ventricle are dilated (Figs. 11–11 and 11–12). As long as the left ventricle functions normally, the left ventricular ejection fraction is increased.

With mitral valve prolapse or ruptured chordae tendineae or papillary muscle, the posterior, and at times the anterior, leaflets prolapse into the left atrium.

Radiographic Features. The radiographic findings correlate well with the hemodynamics and the degree of mitral regurgitation. When the volume of regurgitation is small, the cardiac size and contour and the pulmonary vasculature are normal.

FIGURE 11–12. Mitral insufficiency. M-mode echocardiogram through aorta (Ao) and left atrium (LA). Dilated left atrium. Normally, aortic and left atrial dimensions are identical in this projection.

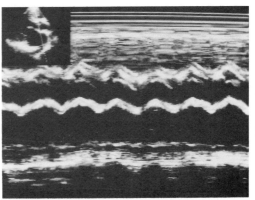

Ao

LA

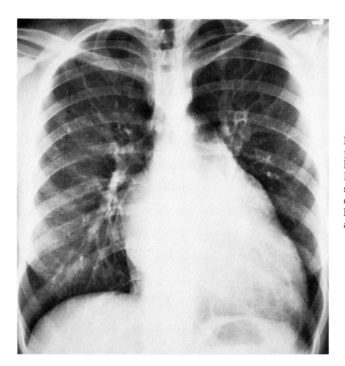

FIGURE 11–13. Mitral insufficiency. Cephalization of vascular markings. Large hilar vessels. Cardiomegaly. Left atrial enlargement is evidenced by a double density, elevation of the left mainstem bronchus, and a large left atrial appendage. Enlargement of the left ventricle laterally and downward.

However, in moderate to severe mitral regurgitation (Figs. 11–13 and 11–14), cardiomegaly is present, principally because of left atrial and left ventricular enlargement. In the posteroanterior projection, left atrial enlargement causes prominence of the left atrial appendage along the left cardiac border, double

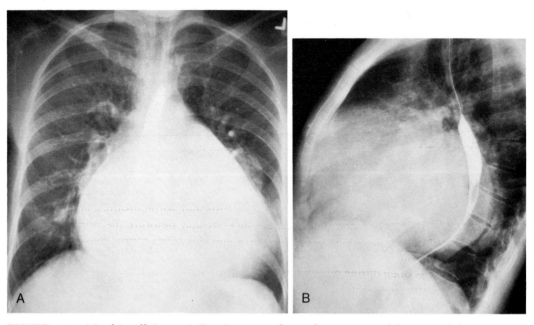

FIGURE 11–14. Mitral insufficiency. A, Prominent vascular markings in upper lobes. Large hilar vessels. Cardiomegaly. Massive dilatation of the left atrium evidenced by double density extending almost across the entire cardiac shadow and by a dilated left atrial appendage. Displacement of the barium-filled esophagus toward right. Right atrial enlargement, evidenced by marked displacement of right cardiac border toward the right. B, Lateral view. Posterior displacement of barium-filled esophagus.

density along the right cardiac border, elevation of the left mainstem bronchus, and displacement of the barium-filled esophagus to the right. In lateral and right anterior oblique projections, left atrial enlargement causes posterior displacement of the mid-portion of the barium-filled esophagus. Left ventricular enlargement alters the cardiac contour by a downward posterior bulge of the left cardiac border in posteroanterior and left anterior oblique projections.

The pulmonary vasculature may show the changes of venous obstruction. Pulmonary blood flow is redistributed to the upper lobes (cephalization). There is pulmonary edema, and there are Kerley B lines in the lower lobes. Eventually, signs of pulmonary arterial hypertension develop: an enlarged pulmonary arterial segment and enlarged central pulmonary arteries that taper rapidly toward the periphery of the lung fields. Right ventricular enlargement develops, causing fullness of the retrosternal space on a lateral projection.

Angiographic Features. Left ventriculography in a 30-degree right anterior oblique projection demonstrates the degree of mitral regurgitation, which is commonly graded on a subjective basis of 1+ to 4+. With 1+ mitral reflux, a well-confined, narrow jet is visualized, and several systoles are required to opacify the left atrium. In 2+ insufficiency, the jet is larger, and more rapid filling of the left atrium occurs. With 3+ regurgitation, there is usually some enlargement of the left ventricle, and either a very large regurgitating jet or no jet may be demonstrated. With 4+ reflux there is invariably left ventricular enlargement, and the left atrium is usually huge.

Management. Symptomatic mitral insufficiency is usually treated by valve replacement but occasionally by mitral valvuloplasty or annuloplasty if there is a discrete lesion or a dilated annulus.

Calcific Valvular Disease

Calcification of the fibrotic annulus of the mitral valve is found in 10 per cent of the hearts of an elderly population. It results from degeneration and is not accompanied by calcification of the valve cusps. It is most easily detected by fluoroscopy or on an over-penetrated film in the lateral projection.

Calcification of the mitral cusps occurs secondary to rheumatic inflammation and accompanies severe mitral stenosis or insufficiency. Calcification of the mitral valve ring or cusps may also be associated with calcific aortic stenosis.

Aortic Valve Disease

Aortic stenosis may be subdivided according to the absence or presence of calcium in the valve cusps. Noncalcific aortic stenosis is almost always caused by rheumatic fever and usually coexists with mitral stenosis and aortic insufficiency. The inflammatory process of rheumatic fever thickens and deforms the aortic valve leaflets. Adhesions develop between the cusps and scar tissue forms, causing thickening and immobility of the cusps. Because the cusps are fused and rigid, they remain partially open during diastole, leading to some degree of regurgitation. Noncalcific aortic stenosis occurs most commonly in individuals younger than 50 years of age and is slightly more common in males.

In contrast, calcific aortic stenosis occurs predominantly in males, presents at a later age, and is often symptomatic. Calcific aortic stenosis usually develops on a congenitally bicuspid aortic valve, and this form is generally associated with post-stenotic dilatation of the ascending aorta. Calcification is uncommon in a rheumatic aortic valve.

Not only are the aortic valve cusps calcified, but so are the sinuses of Valsalva and the fibrotic annulus of the aortic valve. Eventually, the anterior leaflet of the mitral valve and the interventricular septum also become calcified. The coronary ostia are free of atherosclerosis.

Rarely, bacterial endocarditis causes aortic valvular obstruction.

Hemodynamics. In an adult, the orifice of the normal aortic valve is about 3 sq cm. Symptoms appear in patients with a valve orifice less than 0.7 sq cm in isolated aortic stenosis, or of less than 1.5 sq cm in patients with coexistent aortic insufficiency. As a result of the obstruction, a gradient is created between the left ventricle and the aorta that is proportional to the size of the aortic valvular orifice and the volume of flow across it. The degree of stenosis is considered moderate when a gradient of 40 to 50 mm Hg is present; in severe aortic stenosis, the gradient may reach 150 mm Hg. In patients with coexistent aortic regurgitation, the volume of blood flow forward across the valve is increased, and therefore the gradient is larger in relation to the severity of the aortic stenosis.

The principal effect of aortic stenosis is elevation of the left ventricular systolic pressure. This causes left ventricular hypertrophy, which maintains the cardiac output at a normal level. The concentric left ventricular hypertrophy slightly reduces the left ventricular diastolic volume. Left ventricular dilatation is present only in patients with aortic regurgitation or in patients with isolated aortic stenosis as the left ventricle becomes fibrosed and decompensates over decades.

Clinical Features. Angina, syncope, and sudden death are the principal symptoms associated with aortic stenosis and presumably are related to an insufficient oxygen supply to the hypertrophied left ventricular myocardium. These symptoms frequently occur in patients with a normal cardiac size and a large left ventricular–aortic pressure difference. When there is significant aortic regurgitation or extensive myocardial fibrosis, dyspnea and fatigue on exercise may appear, reflecting left ventricular decompensation.

In the aortic area there is a systolic ejection murmur, which is often associated with a thrill. In the same area, an early diastolic murmur is present in patients with coexistent aortic regurgitation. An ejection click is much less common than in patients with congenital aortic valvular stenosis.

The electrocardiogram may be normal, even in patients with moderate stenosis. Signs of left ventricular hypertrophy are expected. In the left precordial leads, the ST segment may become depressed and the T wave inverted, indicating left ventricular strain. This pattern is found in patients with syncope and subsequent sudden death, and its appearance indicates prompt treatment of the cardiac condition.

Echocardiographic Features. On M-mode echocardiography, multiple aortic valve echoes may be seen. During diastole, eccentric closure of the leaflets may be observed when the aortic stenosis results from a congenitally bicuspid valve. The internal dimensions of the ascending aorta may be increased, representing the post-stenotic dilatation. The free left ventricular wall is thickened, generally in proportion to the severity of the stenosis. The internal dimensions of the left ventricle are increased in the presence of aortic regurgitation. These same features may be identified on cross-sectional echocardiography, which better shows the details of the aortic valve leaflets.

Radiographic Features. The radiographic features differ depending on the status of the left ventricle.

In compensated, isolated aortic stenosis, cardiac size is normal (Fig. 11–15). The heart shows a left ventricular contour, with a rounding of the lower left border due to left ventricular hypertrophy. There may also be prominence of the upper right cardiac border if post-stenotic dilatation of the aorta is present. The

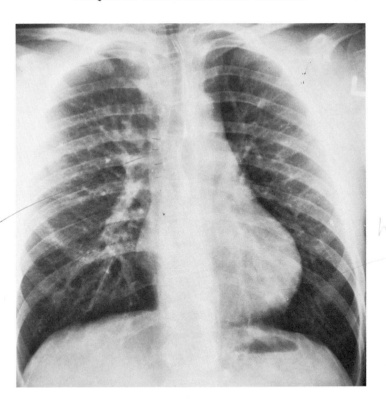

FIGURE 11–15. Compensated aortic stenosis. Normal cardiac size. Round uptilted cardiac apex. Prominent ascending aorta.

pulmonary vasculature is normal. With time the left ventricle dilates and, in addition to the hypertrophy, results in moderate cardiomegaly with a left ventricular configuration (Fig. 11–16).

In decompensated aortic stenosis with significant aortic insufficiency, cardiac

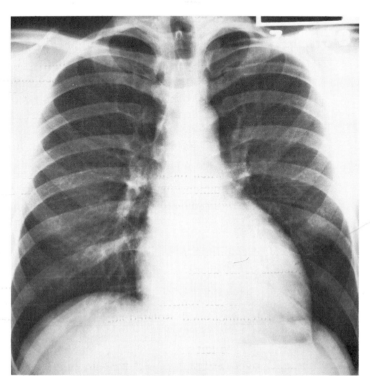

FIGURE 11–16. Aortic stenosis with ventricular dilatation. Normal pulmonary vascularity. Cardiomegaly. Lateral and downward displacement of cardiac apex.

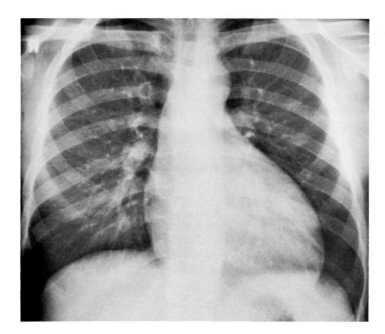

FIGURE 11–17. Decompensated aortic stenosis. Normal pulmonary vascularity. Cardiomegaly. Left ventricular configuration. Prominent ascending aorta and aortic knob.

enlargement is present. The cardiac silhouette has a left ventricular configuration as the left ventricle enlarges posteriorly downward; this enlargement is observed most readily on posteroanterior and left anterior oblique projections (Fig. 11–17). The ascending aorta in bicuspid aortic valves may develop a process of secondary cystic medial degeneration (Fig. 11–18). With cardiac decompensation, radiographic features of left atrial and right ventricular enlargement are found. The lungs eventually show venous obstruction.

Role of Fluoroscopy. Fluoroscopy helps to demonstrate any valvular calcification in patients with aortic stenosis. Calcification of the aortic valve is difficult to demonstrate on chest films unless overpenetrated films are obtained (Fig. 11–18C). Fluoroscopy or cine recording of the valve cusps permits identification of calcification with greater accuracy. Calcification of the fibrotic annulus can be distinguished from calcification of valve cusps, the former being associated with calcium in the form of a ring that shows less pronounced pulsation on fluoroscopy.

Angiographic Appearance. The aortic valve leaflets are thickened and open incompletely during systole. Post-stenotic dilatation is usually minor or absent, contrary to congenital aortic stenosis. (Fig. 11–19). Left ventricular size may be normal.

Management. Calcific aortic stenosis is treated by aortic valve replacement. Occasionally, in adults, a noncalcified valve can be managed by valvotomy.

Aortic Insufficiency

Aortic insufficiency is usually acquired, generally as the result of rheumatic fever. Such rheumatic insufficiency occurs predominaly in males and usually coexists with mitral valvular disease. During the acute phase of rheumatic carditis, the free margins of the valve cusps are inflamed. Subsequently, the cusps scar, becoming too short to close the orifice completely. The aortic annulus may also dilate secondary to rheumatic changes. Such changes may also cause aortic valvular stenosis.

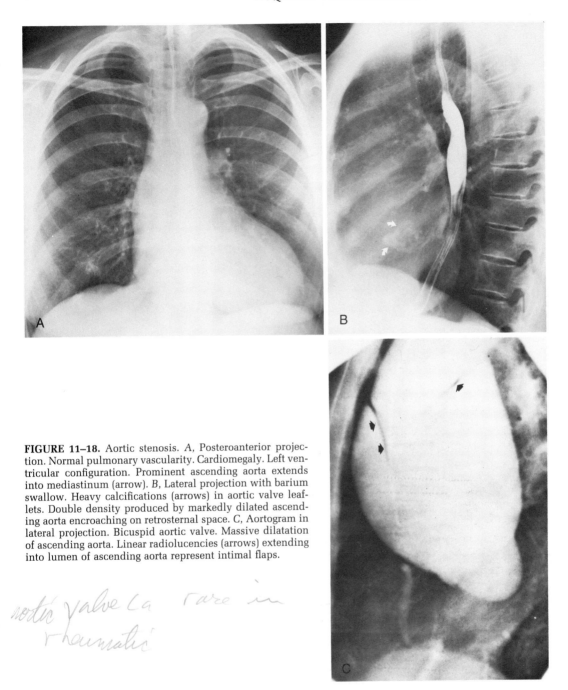

FIGURE 11–18. Aortic stenosis. *A,* Posteroanterior projection. Normal pulmonary vascularity. Cardiomegaly. Left ventricular configuration. Prominent ascending aorta extends into mediastinum (arrow). *B,* Lateral projection with barium swallow. Heavy calcifications (arrows) in aortic valve leaflets. Double density produced by markedly dilated ascending aorta encroaching on retrosternal space. *C,* Aortogram in lateral projection. Bicuspid aortic valve. Massive dilatation of ascending aorta. Linear radiolucencies (arrows) extending into lumen of ascending aorta represent intimal flaps.

Aortic insufficiency can also occur secondary to syphilitic aortitis, which dilates the aortic annulus and the ascending aorta and directly involves and damages the valve leaflets. Another cause is bacterial endocarditis, when vegetations eroding the cusps produce an aneurysm or interfere with closure of the cusps.

Rarely, aortic insufficiency results from direct trauma to the chest, from sudden unusually strenuous muscular exertion, or from dissection of an aortic aneurysm that involves the attachment of aortic cusps. Other rare causes include Marfan's syndrome and collagen diseases, particularly ankylosing spondylitis.

Hemodynamics. The principal hemodynamic effects of aortic insufficiency result from regurgitation of aortic blood into the left ventricle. This regurgitant

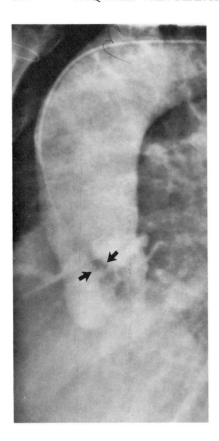

FIGURE 11–19. Aortic stenosis. Aortogram in lateral projection. Aortic insufficiency. Deformity of aortic valve with asymmetric opening and narrow jet (arrows). Minimal dilatation of ascending aorta.

volume plus the normal inflow of blood from the left atrium dilates the left ventricle and increases its diastolic volume. During systole, left ventricular contraction is increased, causing ejection of a larger volume of blood into the aorta (the normal stroke volume plus the regurgitant fraction). Dilatation of the ascending aorta is secondary to the increased volume of blood being ejected into it.

The principal change in the left ventricle is dilatation; hypertrophy occurs as a secondary phenomenon. Usually, the hypertrophy can maintain the additional cardiac volume loads for long periods of time, but eventually left ventricular decompensation develops and leads to congestive cardiac failure. In contrast, when aortic insufficiency develops abruptly, e.g., as the result of trauma or bacterial endocarditis, signs of acute cardiac failure appear.

Clinical Features. Many patients are asymptomatic, but as aortic regurgitation progresses, dyspnea on exertion and fatigue appear. Later the patient has symptoms of cardiac failure. Angina is rare, but severe chest pain may be present in patients with an abrupt onset of aortic regurgitation.

The clinical diagnosis is easy. The pulse pressure is wide, the systolic pressure being elevated by the increased stroke volume and the diastolic pressure being lowered by the runoff of aortic blood into the left ventricle. There is clinical evidence of cardiac enlargement and an active precordium. The major auscultatory finding is an early diastolic murmur along the mid-left sternal border. The louder the murmur, the greater the degree of aortic regurgitation. In patients with a large left ventricular stroke volume, an aortic systolic ejection murmur is heard as well.

The electrocardiogram shows a pattern of left ventricular hypertrophy. With severe aortic insufficiency, the T waves become inverted in the left precordial leads.

Echocardiographic Features. There is dilatation of the left ventricle and ascending aorta. There is a flutter of the anterior leaflet of the mitral valve caused by the regurgitant jet and, occasionally, of the left side of the interventricular septum. There may be echocardiographic findings that suggest the cause of the insufficiency, such as evidence of vegetations on the aortic valve, the mitral prolapse and dilated aortic sinuses of Marfan's syndrome, or mitral valve changes suggesting rheumatic heart disease.

Radiographic Features. The radiographic features vary with the amount of regurgitation. In mild aortic regurgitation, cardiac size is normal, as is the cardiac contour, since slight left ventricular enlargement cannot be recognized. The pulmonary vasculature is normal.

In moderate and severe aortic regurgitation, cardiac enlargement is present,

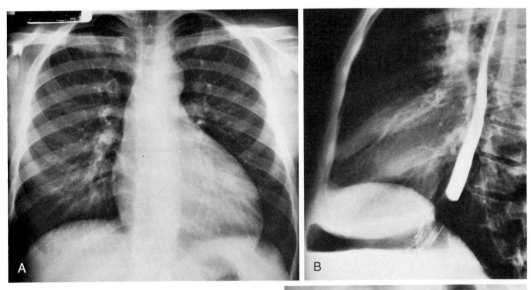

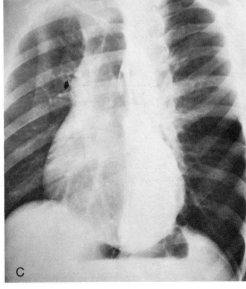

FIGURE 11–20. Aortic insufficiency. *A*, Posteroanterior projection. Normal pulmonary vascularity. Cardiomegaly. Left ventricular configuration. Prominent ascending aorta and aortic knob. *B*, Lateral projection. Marked encroachment on gastric fundus by downward enlargement of left ventricle. *C*, Left anterior oblique projection. The posterior cardiac margin overlaps the spine. Downwardly displaced left ventricle encroaches on gastric fundus. Prominent ascending aorta (arrow).

the size reflecting the regurgitant volume. The cardiac contour shows a left ventricular configuration. The lower left cardiac border is elongated posteriorly and inferiorly and is most easily seen on posteroanterior and left anterior oblique projections (Fig. 11–20). On the latter the left ventricular border may extend beyond the spine (Fig. 11–20C). The enlarged left ventricle displaces the left hemidiaphragm and encroaches on the gastric fundus (Fig. 11–20B); the ascending aorta and aortic knob are dilated because of the post-stenotic dilatation (Fig. 11–20).

In aortic regurgitation with cardiac failure, in addition to the findings described above, there is further dilatation of the left ventricle. The left atrium and pulmonary veins enlarge because of the left ventricular failure and the mitral insufficiency that develops secondary to left ventricular dilatation. The pulmonary vasculature shows a pattern of venous obstruction. Signs of right ventricular and right atrial enlargement may be present if right ventricular failure develops.

In patients with aortic insufficiency of abrupt onset, there is minimal cardiac enlargement and minimal change in the cardiac contour. The pulmonary vasculature shows a prominent pattern of venous obstruction.

Radiographic findings that suggest a particular cause of aortic insufficiency include extensive linear calcification in a dilated ascending aorta (Fig. 11–21) characteristic of syphilitic aortitis, and marked dilatation of the ascending arota (Fig. 11–22) characteristic of Marfan's syndrome.

Angiographic Appearance. Both aortography and left ventriculography should be performed to assess the degree of aortic regurgitation (from 1 + to 4 +) and the status of left ventricular function and myocardial contractility. Hypokinesis is commonly observed in long-standing aortic insufficiency.

Management. In most circumstances, symptomatic aortic insufficiency must be treated by aortic valve replacement, although in an occasional case, aortic valvuloplasty renders the valve competent.

RADIOGRAPHIC IDENTIFICATION OF PROSTHETIC HEART VALVES

Prosthetic cardiac valves can be identified easily from the chest radiograph as to both their location (Fig. 11–23) and their type. Evaluation of valve function can be done only under fluoroscopic observation, either with or without cine recording.

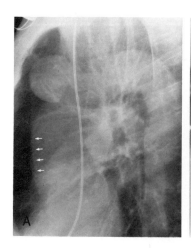 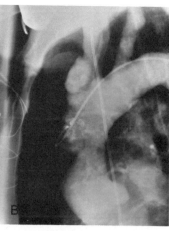

FIGURE 11–21. Aortic insufficiency. A, Dilated ascending aorta with linear calcifications (arrows). Round mass density in upper mediastinum proved to be a thrombosed luetic aneurysm of the brachiocephalic artery. B, Aortogram. No opacification of aneurysm.

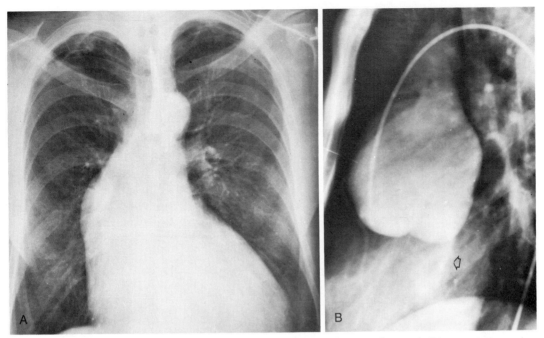

FIGURE 11–22. Aortic insufficiency secondary to Marfan's syndrome. *A,* Posteroanterior projection. Normal pulmonary vascularity. Cardiomegaly with a left ventricular configuration. Large bulge in midsegment of right cardiac margin represents massive dilatation of aortic root and ascending aorta. *B,* Aortogram. Lateral projection. Massive dilatation of sinuses of Valsalva and proximal ascending aorta. Slight degreee of aortic insufficiency (arrow).

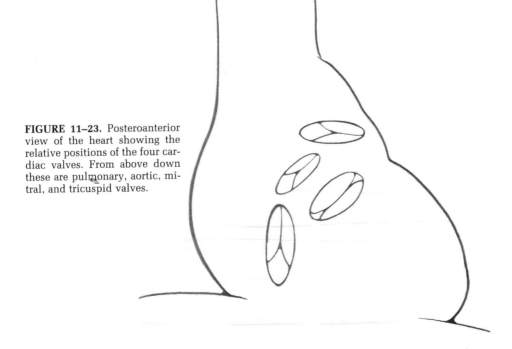

FIGURE 11–23. Posteroanterior view of the heart showing the relative positions of the four cardiac valves. From above down these are pulmonary, aortic, mitral, and tricuspid valves.

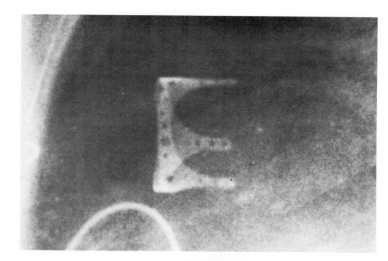

FIGURE 11–24. Ionescu-Shiley xenograft (pulmonary position). Base ring and a stent with many perforations in both.

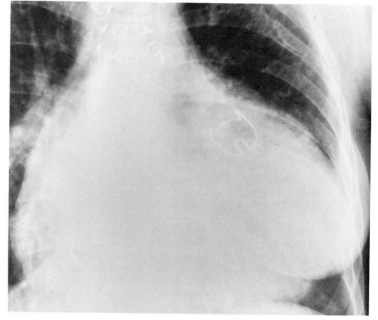

FIGURE 11–25. Edwards xenograft. Serpentine-like radiopaque wire stent. Base ring is radiolucent.

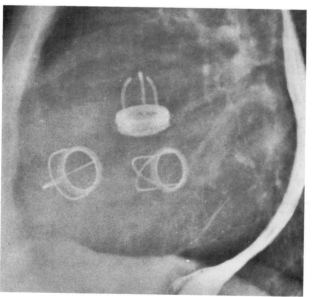

FIGURE 11–26. Magovern-Cromie prosthesis (aortic position). Three struts from the cage, which has a large apical opening. Nonradiopaque ball. Starr-Edwards prostheses in tricuspid and mitral positions.

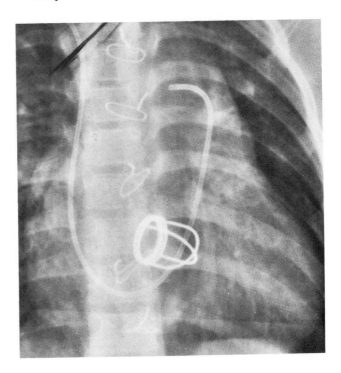

FIGURE 11–27. Starr-Edwards prosthesis (mitral position). Four struts form closed cage around radiolucent ball. No notch at strut-base ring junction. Base ring has single encircling groove.

The radiographic identification of the specific type of prosthetic heart valves is made from the observation of the following components of the valve: base ring, stent, ball or disk, and cage and struts. Prosthetic heart valves are of two major types: mechanical and heterograft.

Heterograft prostheses can be distinguished from mechanical valves by

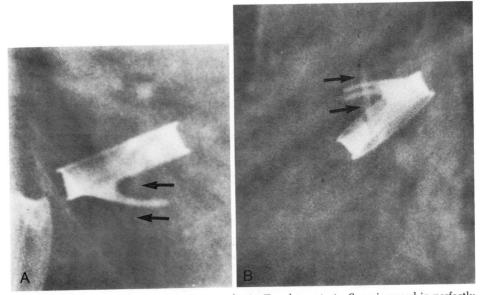

FIGURE 11–28. *A,* Lillehei-Kaster valve prosthesis. Two large struts. Superimposed in perfectly tangential view of valve, to facilitate the demonstration of the valve disc (arrows). Base ring is clearly seen. *B,* Lillehei-Kaster valve prosthesis in aortic position. Valve disc is better seen in open position (arrows). Two struts are well seen because of an incomplete superimposition during radiographic projection.

observation of the base ring. In a heterograft valve there is only a base ring and it can be identified easily (Fig. 11–24). The only other structure that might be radiopaque in the heterograft prosthesis is the stent (Figs. 11–24 and 11–25).

Mechanical valve prostheses may be divided into two large groups, either

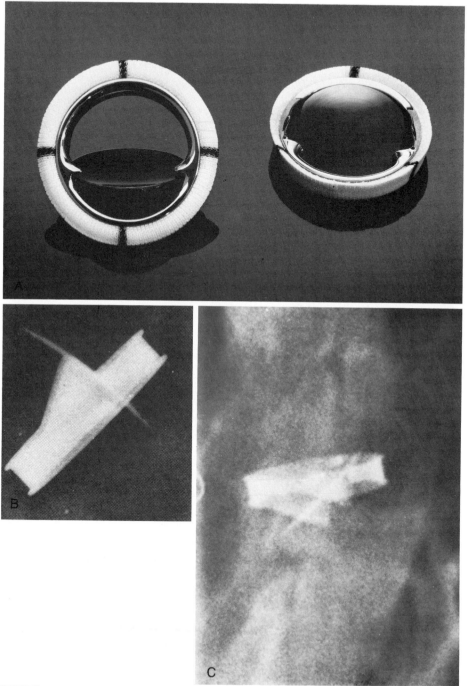

FIGURE 11–29. A, Omniscience valve prosthesis in open (left) and closed (right) positions. B, Omniscience valve. Two short triangular-shaped struts emerge from base ring. Radiopaque disk seen during opening. C, Incomplete superimposition of struts. Disk clearly seen. Valve in mitral position.

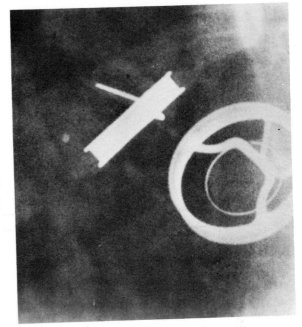

FIGURE 11–30. Bjork-Shiley valve prosthesis in mitral and aortic positions. Base ring encircled by groove. From base ring two eccentrically placed U-shaped structures of unequal size emerge. Radiolucent disk; radiopaque ring surrounds disk. Aortic prosthesis is seen in perfectly tangential view, demonstrating complete opening of valve disk. Mitral prosthesis seen on end, allowing visualization of disk and two U-shaped retainers.

high or low profile valves. The examination of the valve cage and of the mobile portion of the valve allows the differentiation between these two types. In a high profile mechanical prosthesis the mobile portion of the valve is a ball, which is usually nonopaque or barely radiopaque (Figs. 11–26 and 11–27). In a low profile prosthesis, the mobile portion is a disk. In a high profile prosthesis, the cage is taller than the cage of a low profile prosthesis, since it must accommodate the movements of the ball. Only the most commonly used mechanical prostheses are illustrated in this chapter.

To identify the different low profile valve prostheses, the number and morphology of the struts should be determined and the features of the valve disk

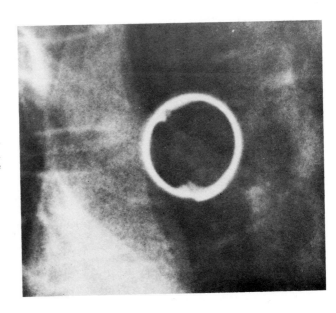

FIGURE 11–31. A, Wada-Cutter prosthesis. Two eccentrically placed notched projections of equal size emerge from base ring. Disk is radiolucent.

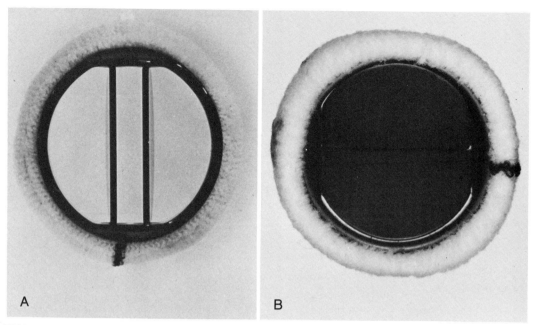

FIGURE 11–32. St. Jude's valve prosthesis in open (A) and closed (B) positions.

evaluated (Figs. 11–28 and 11–29). The valve disk in the Bjork-Shiley (Fig. 11–30) and the Wada-Cutter (Fig. 11–31) is nonopaque. Sometimes they can have a visible ring. The disk in a St. Jude's valve is represented by two halves that move synchronously (Figs. 11–32 and 11–33A and B). The half disks can be observed

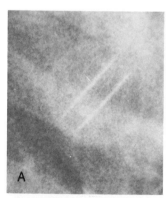

FIGURE 11–33. St. Jude's valve prosthesis. Valve is barely radiopaque. To visualize two halves of disk they must be perfectly on end. A, St. Jude's prosthesis on end, base ring faintly seen. Two half disks seen during complete opening. B and C, St. Jude's prosthesis in profile. Two half disks seen closed (B) and open (C).

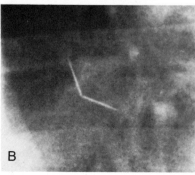

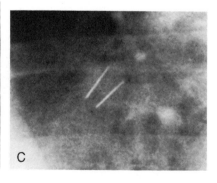

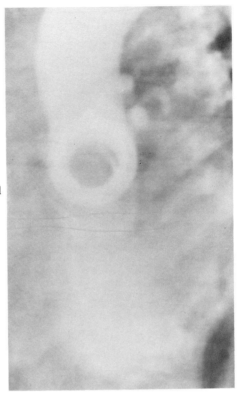

FIGURE 11–34. Magovern valve prosthesis partially detached from suture line. Massive reflux into left ventricle.

from a tangential plane (Fig. 11–33C), or the valve ring can be seen on end, in which case both half disks will be seen on end (Fig. 11–33A).

Once the type of valve is identified, its function is evaluated under fluoroscopic observation with or without cine recording. Two aspects of function are observed. The motion of the valve ring is studied, since this can provide information about partial detachment of the valve ring from its insertion in cardiac tissue. When this occurs, there is asymmetric movement of the valve ring (Fig. 11–34).

The movement of the valve disk is the second functional aspect observed. Development of thrombus is the most common cause of valve malfunctioning. The valve disk should be observed tangentially and its angle of opening measured (Figs. 11–28, 11–30 and 11–33).

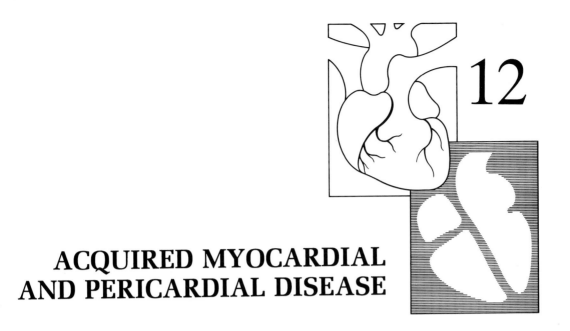

ACQUIRED MYOCARDIAL AND PERICARDIAL DISEASE

CONGESTIVE CARDIAC FAILURE

Congestive cardiac failure is difficult to define exactly. It occurs when the heart fails to maintain an adequate circulation for the needs of the body despite a satisfactory venous filling pressure. Clinically, the term denotes a set of signs and symptoms secondary to fluid retention and venous congestion.

Congestive cardiac failure is not a disease state, but rather the consequence of a severe underlying condition that places abnormal workloads on the heart or alters the contractile response of the myocardium. The causes of congestive cardiac failure may be classified as:

1. Abnormality of the myocardium. Myocardial infarction and cardiomyopathies are two types of disease that decrease myocardial contractility. Congestive cardiac failure commonly develops in patients with myocardial diseases.

2. Increased left ventricular volume. Conditions such as severe anemia, mitral or aortic regurgitation, ventricular septal defect, or patent ductus arteriosus are commonly associated with congestive cardiac failure. Because the left ventricle is conical, increased volume loads can be accommodated only by left ventricular dilatation. Because the left ventricle develops a high systolic pressure when it dilates, the amount of tension necessary to maintain the cardiac output eventually reaches excessive levels. Cardiac failure then results.

3. Increased left ventricular systolic pressure. Aortic stenosis can be well tolerated for decades because the shape and musculature of the left ventricle are suitable for the production of increased pressure. However, if myocardial fibrosis develops in the left ventricle, left ventricular failure occurs.

4. Increased right ventricular systolic pressure, e.g., in patients with cor pulmonale. The normal right ventricle is thin-walled and has a large radius and a low pressure. With even modest increases in right ventricular systolic pressure, the right ventricle cannot generate sufficient tension to create that pressure and cardiac failure appears.

5. Increased right ventricular volume, e.g., in tricuspid insufficiency or atrial septal defect. Usually, this condition is well tolerated; cardiac failure appears only if the volume load is excessive or of long duration. The explanation lies in the

fact that the right ventricle can alter its shape to accommodate a larger volume of blood without stretching its myofibrils and the right ventricular systolic pressure is low.

Because either side of the heart may have anomalies, the clinical picture of cardiac failure has been divided into two types. In left-sided cardiac failure, the principal signs and symptoms are related to engorgement of the pulmonary veins and capillaries. In right-sided cardiac failure, the principal signs and symptoms are related to engorgement of the systemic veins and capillaries.

There are a number of compensatory circulatory responses that tend to maintain adequate circulation. However, as the disease progresses, these compensatory mechanisms may no longer be adequate and, in fact, may eventually become deleterious.

The first of these compensatory responses is cardiac dilatation. According to Starling's law, when the myocardial fibers stretch, cardiac function increases. This is true only to a particular level beyond which continued elongation of myocardial fibers is associated with decreased cardiac function. Thus, dilatation is initially advantageous but eventually becomes disadvantageous.

The second compensatory response is cardiac hypertrophy. As the ventricle dilates and tension in its wall increases, hypertrophy develops. However, as the fibers hypertrophy, the distance that oxygen must diffuse to reach the center of the fiber increases; this hypoxia may lead to fibrosis in the myocardium.

The third compensatory response is increased sympathetic tone leading eventually to tachycardia and systemic arteriolar constriction. Another mechanism is a regional redistribution of blood flow arising from the renal and splanchnic beds that tends to preserve coronary and cerebral flow. This leads in turn to salt and water retention as a result of decreased glomerular filtration and increased tubular reabsorption.

Finally, there is an elevation of the venous pressure. In left-sided failure, when the left atrial pressure reaches 25 to 30 mm Hg, the hydrostatic pressure in pulmonary capillaries exceeds the osmotic pressure of plasma proteins, and fluid leaves the capillaries and enters the alveoli. Because there is also fluid in the alveolar walls and the pulmonary venous pressure is elevated, the lungs are less compliant. In right-sided failure, elevated venous pressure causes hepatomegaly, and, when the pressure reaches 25 to 30 mm Hg, peripheral edema appears.

Left-Heart Failure

The most common causes of left-sided failure are myocardial infarction, systemic hypertension, cardiomyopathy, aortic stenosis, and mitral insufficiency. The principal clinical features are those of pulmonary congestion, with either dyspnea on exertion or acute pulmonary edema. On examination, tachypnea, rales, and the features of the underlying cardiac condition are found.

Radiographic Features. Radiographically, the earliest manifestation of heart failure is indistinctness of the pulmonary vascular markings as a result of the presence of increased amounts of interstitial fluid, especially at the lung bases (see Fig. 4-40). Later, "cephalization" occurs; i.e., the vascular markings are prominent in the upper lobes because of the constriction of the lower-lobe vessels and consequent redistribution of flow to the upper lobes (see Fig. 4-41). The hilar vessels become enlarged and indistinct. The increased interstitial fluid can also be seen around the cross sections of the bronchi as "peribronchial cuffing" (see Fig. 4-36). Pleural effusion occurs late and is more prominent on the right side than on the left side. Cardiac size is almost invariably increased in heart failure (see Fig. 4–42).

If fluid is transudated into the alveoli, the result is pulmonary edema. Characteristically, this is perihilar, creating a radiographic appearance called "butterfly wings" or "bat wings" (see Fig. 4–43). The peripheral lung fields are usually clear except in severe cases when the lung fields are entirely consolidated (see Fig. 4–43). Kerley B lines are also seen in pulmonary edema (see Fig. 4–41A).

Although pulmonary edema classically involves both lungs, unilateral or focal pulmonary edema can occur if the interstitial or hydrostatic pressure differs in the two lungs. Examples of this phenomenon are seen in patients with orthostatic unilateral pulmonary edema (see Fig. 4–44) or with obstructive pulmonary disease with areas of focal edema in the remaining functioning pulmonary tissue (see Fig. 4–45).

Right-Heart Failure

The most common causes of right-heart failure are left ventricular failure, cor pulmonale, and tricuspid insufficiency. The clinical features are engorged neck veins, hepatomegaly, and ankle edema.

Radiographic Features. Often, there is left ventricular enlargement so that the entire heart is enlarged. In cor pulmonale, there are characteristic pulmonary vascular changes, depending on the underlying condition (Chapter 12). When right-heart failure is secondary to chronic lung disease, the lungs are hyperaerated and the hemidiaphragms are low.

Management. Management of congestive heart failure is medical: bed rest to reduce cardiac output, digitalis to increase myocardial contractility, and diuretics to promote fluid loss. Afterload reducing agents—drugs that lower systemic vascular resistance—have recently been successful in increasing cardiac output in patients with left-heart failure.

Selected Bibliography

Artman, M., Parrish, M. D., and Graham, T.: Congestive heart failure in childhood and adolescence: Recognition and management. Am. Heart J., *105*(3):471–480, 1983.

Perloff, J. K.: The clinical manifestations of cardiac failure in adults. Hosp. Pract., 2:43–50, 1970.

Talner, N. S.: The pathophysiology of congestive heart failure in infancy. Pediatr. Cardiol., *1*:120–136, 1979.

CARDIOMYOPATHY

Cardiomyopathies are a broad group of anomalies of various origins having three features in common.

1. Failure of the heart to maintain the cardiac output. This results in features of cardiac failure and inadequate perfusion.

2. Failure of the heart to maintain its architecture. Cardiomegaly and often mitral insufficiency develop because of dilatation of the cardiac chambers.

3. Failure of the heart to maintain the electrical activity. There are frequently ST/T wave changes and arrhythmias.

The origin of cardiomyopathies is diverse and includes (1) infections, particularly viral, causing myocarditis; (2) metabolic diseases involving storage of abnormal materials such as glycogen or carnitine; (3) skeletal muscle diseases—in many patients with cardiomyopathy, histologic abnormalities are also present in skeletal muscle; (4) cardiotoxic agents such as those used for malignancies; and (5) familial.

In cardiomyopathies myocardial function is abnormal; principally left ventricle contractility is decreased and the left ventricle is dilated. Both the cardiac output and ejection fraction are decreased. Left ventricular end-diastolic pressure is usually elevated, and this leads to the elevation of pulmonary venous pressure. Because of left ventricular dilatation, mitral insufficiency may develop, further increasing left ventricular volume and end-diastolic pressure.

Clinical Features. Regardless of the etiology of the cardiomyopathy, the symptoms are similar. Dyspnea and fatigue on exertion are the major symptoms. Subsequently there are other features of cardiac failure. Angina or lightheadedness may be described and these indicate an inadequate cardiac output.

On examination, there is often a precordial bulge and the cardiac apex is displaced laterally and inferiorly. There may be either no murmur or a soft murmur of mitral insufficiency. A gallop rhythm is common.

The electrocardiogram may show a pattern of left ventricular hypertrophy. ST segment depression and T wave inversion are observed in the left precordial leads.

Echocardiographic Features. The internal dimensions of the left ventricle are increased (Figs. 12–1 and 12–2) and show little change between systole

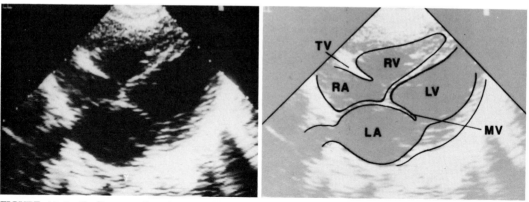

FIGURE 12–1. Cardiomyopathy. Cross-sectional echocardiogram. Apical four-chamber view. Dilated left ventricle (LV). TV, Tricuspid valve; RV, right ventricle; RA, right atrium; LA, left atrium; MV, mitral valve.

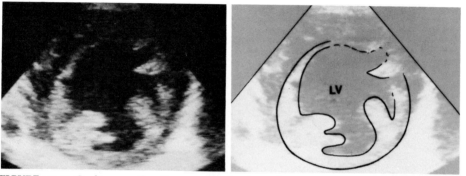

FIGURE 12–2. Cardiomyopathy. Cross-sectional echocardiogram. Short axis-view. Dilated left ventricle (LV).

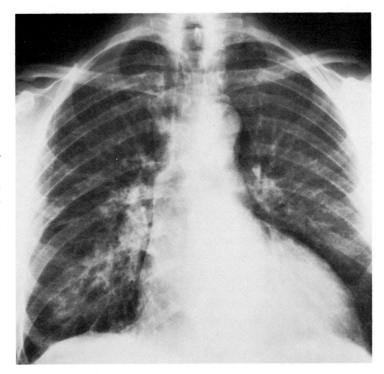

FIGURE 12–3. Cardiomyopathy. Thoracic roentgenogram. Postero-anterior projection. Cardiomegaly with a left ventricular configuration. Lateral displacement of cardiac apex. Indistinct vascular markings in lower lobes. Redistribution of blood flow toward upper lobes.

and diastole. The left ventricular posterior wall is usually of normal thickness. The movements of the mitral valve may be diminished because of reduced flow through it.

Radiographic Features (Fig. 12–3)

1. There is generalized cardiac enlargement.

2. The cardiac apex is displaced downward and to the left because of the left ventricular enlargement.

3. The left cardiac border shows a broad, round contour of left ventricular enlargement.

4. Left atrial enlargement is common.

5. The pulmonary vasculature may be normal or show a pattern of pulmonary venous obstruction.

Management. Cardiomyopathies are usually progressive and intractable. Digitalis, diuretics, and afterload reducing agents are the principal drugs used.

Selected Bibliography

Lerner, A. M., Wilson, F. M., and Reyes, M. P.: Enteroviruses and the heart (with special emphasis on the probable role of coxsackieviruses, group B, types 1-5). II. Observations in humans. Mod. Concepts Cardiovasc. Dis., *44*(3):11–18, 1975.
Perloff, J. K.: The cardiomyopathies: Dilated and restrictive. (Key References). Circulation, *63*(5):1189–1198, 1981.

HYPERTENSIVE CARDIOVASCULAR DISEASE

Systemic hypertension affects many people and is a leading cause of death in the United States. Death results from the effects of hypertension on the cerebral, renal, and coronary arteries, and from the increased workload on the left ventricle.

Definition of systemic hypertension is difficult, but blood pressure levels above 140/90 mm Hg are generally considered hypertensive for adults.

The blood pressure is determined principally by cardiac output and peripheral arteriolar resistance. Blood pressure varies even in an individual and depends on factors such as the level of activity and anxiety. At rest, cardiac output is at its lowest, so hypertension at rest is usually caused by changes in peripheral resistance.

Indeed, systemic hypertension is principally a disease of increased peripheral arteriolar resistance rather than abnormal cardiac output. In some patients, identifiable causes, such as acute or chronic renal disease, certain diseases of the adrenal gland, and particular cerebral lesions are identified. In most patients, however, no identifiable cause is found, although excessive intake of sodium, stress, anxiety, lack of exercise, and a family history of hypertension are relevant factors.

Initially, hypertension is believed to result from increased peripheral arteriolar resistance secondary to vasoconstriction. Changes in the structure of the arterioles lead to fixed narrowing; thus systemic hypertension tends to propagate itself. The increased systemic blood pressure causes left ventricular hypertrophy. Eventually, left ventricular failure and dilatation may occur as fibrosis develops in the left ventricle. The fibrosis develops in part because of an imbalance between myocardial oxygen supply and demand, the oxygen supply being limited by coronary atherosclerosis that develops in response to systemic hypertension. Hypertension also accelerates atherosclerosis in the systemic arteries, and serious symptoms and signs result from impairment in the cerebral, renal, and coronary arteries.

Clinical Features. Most patients with hypertension are asymptomatic. The first symptoms are often related to complications of the condition such as stroke, angina, myocardial infarction, or left ventricular failure.

The diagnosis is made by taking a blood pressure reading. There may be a left ventricular heave. Often a soft aortic ejection murmur is present and later a short diastolic murmur of aortic insufficiency. A fourth heart sound may be present.

The electrocardiogram is normal in patients with slightly elevated blood pressure, but a pattern of left ventricular hypertrophy is present in many patients with more serious disease. ST and T wave changes appear in patients with severe stenosis or coronary atherosclerosis.

Echocardiographic Features. Initially, the echocardiogram shows symmetrical thickening of the left ventricle. Subsequently, when the left ventricle dilates its internal diameter is increased.

Radiographic Features. In mild hypertension, the chest radiograph is normal. In moderate or long-standing hypertension, cardiac size is initially normal and the cardiac silhouette shows a left ventricular configuration. Later, cardiac enlargement develops and eventually a pulmonary venous congestion is present.

Management. In patients with hypertension from an identifiable cause such as coarctation of the aorta, renovascular anomalies, or pheochromocytoma, the lesion can be treated surgically. In most instances, since no cause is found, treatment is usually directed to lowering the blood pressure and includes weight loss, sodium restriction, and treatment with antihypertensive drugs, of which there is a wide variety in terms of pharmacologic actions and effectiveness. In most patients, the blood pressure can be brought into the normal range with medical management.

Selected Bibliography

Brown, J. J., Fraser, R., Lever, A. F., and Robertson, J. I. S.: Hypertension: A review of selected topics. World Med., *45*(9):549–644, 1971 (Abstract).

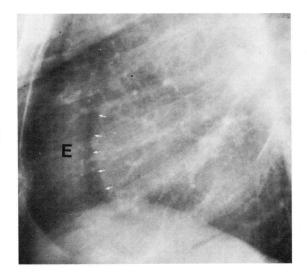

FIGURE 12–7. Acute pericarditis. Thoracic roentgenogram in lateral projection. Radiolucent line (fat pad) separates cardiac silhouette in two parts (arrows), pericardial effusion (E) (front) and cardiac shadow (behind).

2. The cardiac contour shows no demarcation of the chambers or great vessels.

3. The cardiac contour has been described as a waterbottle.

4. The pulmonary vascularity is normal.

5. Cardiac fluoroscopy shows decreased or absent pulsations. However, in cardiac failure and with myopathies, the pulsations are also decreased.

6. Pericardial fat-pad sign (Fig. 12–7).

Pericardial Tamponade

Pericardial tamponade is a physiologic state resulting from either excessive pericardial effusion or pericardial scarring in which cardiac filling is impeded. With the accumulation of large amounts of pericardial fluid or with constriction of the pericardium, the ventricles cannot expand adequately during diastole. This limitation of diastolic filling of the ventricle causes an increase in pulmonary and systemic venous pressures and a fall in cardiac output and decrease in pulse pressure. There is tachycardia and weak arterial pulses.

There are no distinctive radiographic fetures.

Chronic Constrictive Pericarditis

Tuberculosis was formerly the most common cause of constrictive pericarditis. Now, constrictive pericarditis is an uncommon problem; it may occur as a late complication of acute pericarditis of infectious or neoplastic origin, or following intrapericardial hemorrhage. The pericardium becomes thickened and fibrous and it may calcify.

Because of the pericardial scarring the ventricles cannot distend during diastole. The hemodynamics of cardiac tamponade result. Some patients develop protein-losing enteropathy, probably from increased inferior vena caval and portal venous pressure causing increased interstitial capillary pressure and distention of intestinal lymphatics, so that protein is lost into the intestinal lumen.

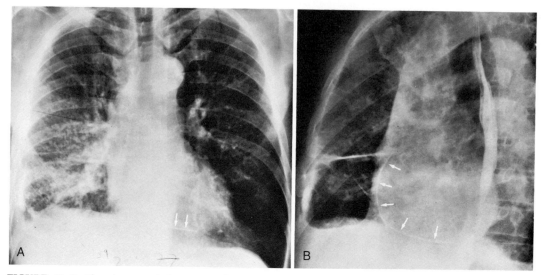

FIGURE 12–8. Chronic constrictive pericarditis. Thoracic roentgenograms. *A,* Posteroanterior projection. Extensive pleural thickening on right. Diffuse nodularity in mid and lower right lung field. Normal cardiac size. Linear density (arrows) along lower cardiac silhouette. *B,* Left anterior oblique projection. Pleural scarring in right lung. Extensive linear calcifications (arrows) surrounding anterior and inferior margins of cardiac silhouette.

Radiographic Features

1. Cardiac size is normal or small. Occasionally it is enlarged because of pre-existing cardiac disease.

2. A rim of calcification may be seen in the pericardium in 50 per cent of patients. The presence of calcification does not imply constriction (Fig. 12–8).

3. Occasionally there is straightening of the right atrial border and rarely of the left cardiac border.

4. On fluoroscopy, cardiac pulsations may be diminished, and this may be either localized or generalized. In many cases the pulsations are normal.

Management. Treatment of pericarditis is largely symptomatic and involves administration of anti-inflammatory agents. Purulent pericarditis is an emergency that requires drainage of the pericardial sac, preferably through a small thoracotomy rather than simply pericardiocentesis, and the administration of large amounts of antibiotics.

Asymptomatic pericardial effusion does not usually require treatment. Pericardial effusion and tamponade require immediate pericardiocentesis to relieve the impaired ventricular filling.

Chronic constrictive pericarditis is treated by surgical removal of the pericardium.

Pericardial Defect

This is a rare condition affecting the pericardium that causes characteristic radiographic findings.

Congenital anomalies such as total absence or defect of the pericardium are uncommon. The cardiac contour is abnormal. A localized defect in the pericardium is located along the left cardiac border through which the left atrial appendage may herniate, causing a characteristic radiographic pattern (Fig. 12–9). The atrial appendage may strangulate.

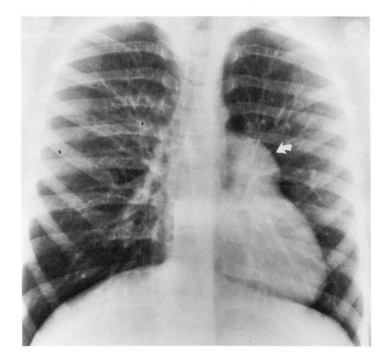

FIGURE 12–9. Partial absence of the pericardium. Thoracic roentgenogram. Posteroanterior projection. Normal pulmonary vascularity. Normal cardiac size. Bulge along left upper cardiac border represents herniated left atrial appendage (arrow).

Selected Bibliography

Anaud, S. S., Saini, V. K., and Wahi, P. L.: Constrictive pericarditis. Dis. Chest, *47*:291, 1961.

Jorgens, J., Blank, N., and Wilcox, W. A.: The cinefluorographic detection and recording of calcifications within the heart: Results of 803 examinations. Radiology, *74*:550, 1960.

Moss, A. J., and Bruhn, F.: The echocardiogram. An ultrasound technic for the detection of pericardial effusion. N. Engl. J. Med., *274*:380–384, 1966.

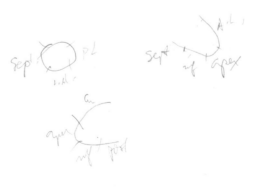

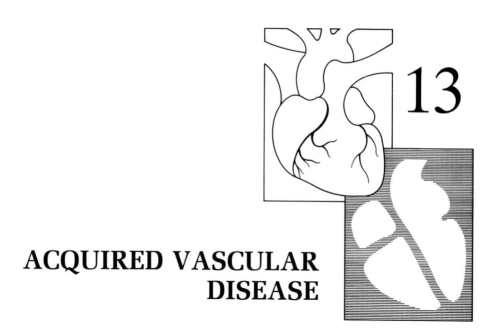

ACQUIRED VASCULAR DISEASE

CORONARY ANGIOGRAPHY

Anatomy of the Coronary Vessels

Right Coronary Artery (Figs. 13–1 to 13–3). The right coronary artery arises immediately above the right aortic sinus and passes anteriorly to the right. It courses between the pulmonary artery and right atrium to enter the right

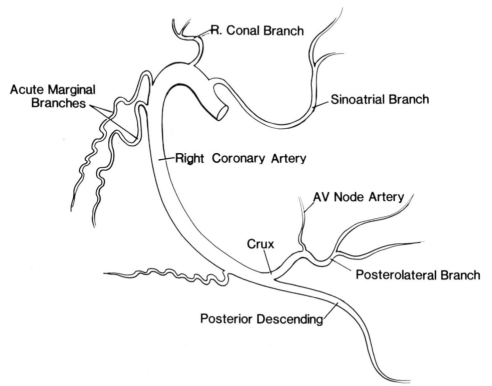

FIGURE 13–1. The right coronary artery in left anterior oblique projection with cephalad angulation. Note that the crux is well seen.

233

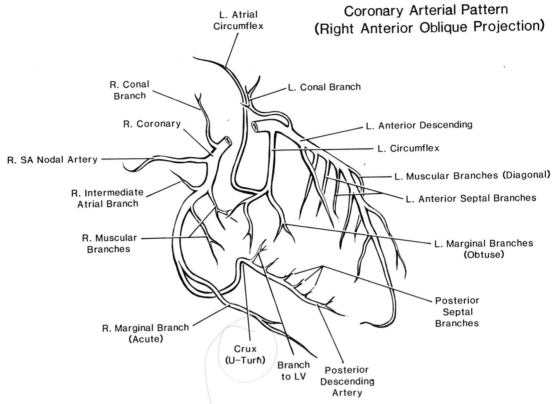

FIGURE 13–2. Right and left coronary arteries in the right anterior oblique projection.

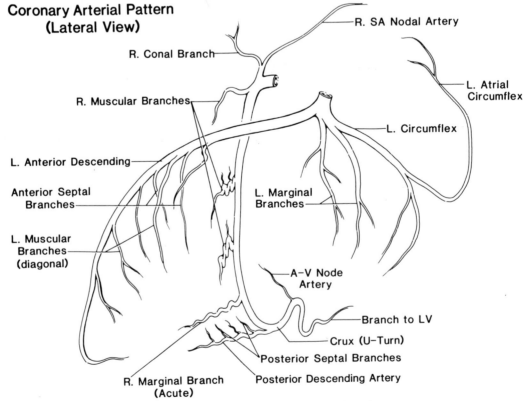

FIGURE 13–3. Right and left coronary arteries in lateral projection.

atrioventricular sulcus. It then passes along the right atrioventricular sulcus past the acute margin of the heart to the base of the posterior interventricular sulcus, the crux.

In 10 per cent of patients, the right coronary artery terminates at the crux. More commonly, the right coronary artery makes a sharp **U**-turn and continues toward the cardiac apex as the posterior descending coronary artery.

The right coronary artery has several major branches. If the conus artery does not arise directly from the aorta as a separate artery, it is the first branch of the right coronary artery and supplies the right ventricular infundibulum. In about 55 per cent of patients, the next major branch arising from the right coronary artery is the sinus node artery, which passes posteriorly to the right atrial appendage and proceeds upward toward the junction of the superior vena cava and the right atrium. In its course, it supplies branches to the right atrium.

The mid-right atrial branch arises past the origin of the sinus nodes artery.

Two or more muscular branches arise from the right coronary artery to the free wall of the right ventricle—some passing to the inferior wall of the right ventricle. The acute marginal branch is the largest branch of the right coronary artery and runs along the acute margin of the right ventricle. It supplies the anterior and diaphragmatic walls of the right ventricle.

In most cases, the right coronary artery terminates by dividing into two branches, the posterior descending and the posterolateral ventricular branches. The latter courses for varying distances in the left atrioventricular sulcus and then descends over the lateral wall of the left ventricle, where it terminates.

Left Coronary Artery (Figs. 13–2 to 13–4). The left coronary artery arises above the left aortic sinus and passes toward the left under the left atrial

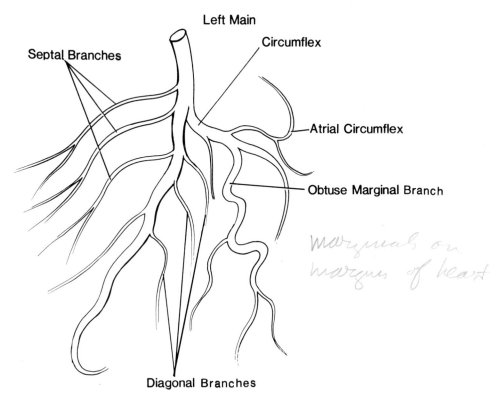

FIGURE 13–4. Left coronary artery in left anterior oblique projection with cephalad angulation.

appendage. After a short course (0.5 to 1.5 cm), the left coronary artery divides into two vessels, the left anterior descending coronary artery and the circumflex artery. In exceptional cases, the left coronary artery trifurcates and gives rise to the left anterior descending, circumflex, and diagonal branches.

The left anterior descending coronary artery passes into the anterior interventricular sulcus, usually as a direct continuation of the left main coronary artery, and extends toward the cardiac apex. Occasionally, it may cross the apex and terminate in the posterior interventricular sulcus. The branches of the left anterior descending artery are the septal branches that penetrate the interventricular septum anteriorly, and one or more diagonal branches. The first diagonal branch is usually larger; its width may be equal to that of the left anterior descending coronary artery.

A left conus branch of the left anterior descending artery may arise near the origin of the first septal branch and proceed toward the right ventricular infundibulum.

The circumflex artery arises at a sharp angle from the left coronary artery and curves under the left atrial appendage to enter the left atrioventricular sulcus.

The course of the circumflex artery is variable. In some instances, the artery gives rise to a large obtuse marginal branch that runs from the atrioventricular sulcus toward the cardiac apex along the lateral wall of the left ventricle. In these cases, the circumflex artery beyond this point is small. In other instances, the circumflex artery, after giving rise to one or more obtuse marginal branches, continues in the left atrioventricular sulcus and terminates near the crux. The circumflex artery continues as the posterior descending artery arises from the right coronary artery.

Veins of the Heart. There are two major groups of coronary veins. One is composed of veins that accompany the major arteries. These are epicardial veins that drain into the coronary sinus. The other group is known collectively as the thebesian system and comprises a variable number of small veins that open directly into the atria.

The course of the coronary sinus parallels the circumflex artery and lies in the left atrioventricular sulcus, entering the posterior aspect of the right atrium. The major tributaries of the coronary sinus are the anterior interventricular vein, the posterior interventricular vein, and the left marginal vein. Opacification of epicardial cardiac veins may be observed in the late phases of coronary arteriograms.

Techniques of Selective Coronary Arteriography

In 1959, Sones described a technique for selective coronary arteriography through a brachial arterial approach. Several types of catheters for selective catheterization of the coronary arteries and different techniques were subsequently developed. Of all the techniques available, two, the Amplatz and the Judkins techniques, are the most widely used.

Amplatz Technique. In 1966, Amplatz described his technique of transfemoral catheterization of the coronary arteries, using a differently shaped catheter for each coronary artery. The catheter for the left coronary artery has a primary curve that is advanced against the aortic valve leaflets. This causes a gradual upward motion of the catheter tip toward the ostium of the left coronary artery. The right coronary artery catheter has a different primary curvature and a secondary curve that conforms to the aortic arch, facilitating the anterior rotation toward the orifice of the right coronary artery.

Judkins Technique. Individually shaped catheters are used for the selective catheterization of the coronary arteries. While the left coronary artery catheter commonly enters by itself into the ostium of the left coronary artery, the right must be manipulated in the same fashion as the right coronary catheter of the Amplatz technique.

Radiographic Technique

Magnification and axial angulation of the x-ray beam with a multidirectional unit are necessary for adequate visualization of the different segments of both coronary arteries. Biplane cine recording is helpful because it decreases the number of injections.

Radiographic Projections

Ten radiographic projections are commonly used to visualize the coronary arteries. Each projection demonstrates different segments of the coronary arteries. Some or all of these projections may be necessary for demonstration of the anatomy of the different segments of the coronary arteries. Depending on the location of the lesions, one or more projections may be either added or deleted.

Left Coronary Artery (Figs. 13–5 and 13–6)

Ten projections may be used to visualize the left coronary artery.

Anteroposterior without Beam Angulation. This is an excellent projection for the visualization of the left main coronary artery. This artery is better visualized using a shallow (5 to 10 degree) left anterior obliquity. The proximal left anterior descending (LAD) is foreshortened in the anteroposterior projection, but the intermediate and distal segments of the LAD and the origin of the second, third, and fourth diagonal arteries are well visualized. The proximal segment of the

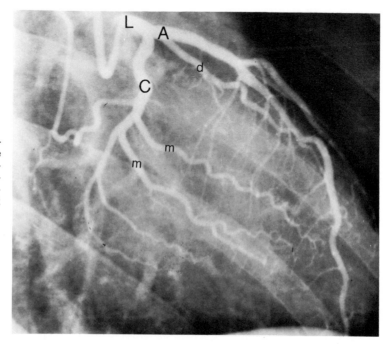

FIGURE 13–5. Left coronary angiogram in right anterior oblique projection with caudad angulation. Circumflex (C) obtuse marginals (m). Left anterior descending artery (A). Diagonals (d). Left main (L).

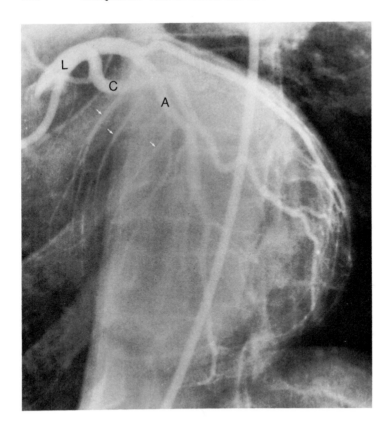

FIGURE 13–6. Left coronary angiogram in left anterior oblique projection. Septal branches (arrows) to the left of the left anterior descending branch (A). L, left coronary artery; C, circumflex branch.

circumflex artery is foreshortened, but its distal segment and marginal branches are well demonstrated.

Anteroposterior with Cephalad Angulation. This view eliminates the overlapping of the first diagonal artery and the proximal left anterior descending coronary artery, thereby facilitating the demonstration of lesions in these arteries. This projection, however, increases the foreshortening of the proximal portion of the circumflex artery.

Anteroposterior with Caudad Angulation. This projection provides a superb demonstration of the bifurcation of the left main coronary into its two major branches, the left anterior descending and circumflex arteries. The proximal and middle segments of the circumflex artery are well seen, since foreshortening is eliminated. The left anterior descending and diagonal branches are also excellently demonstrated in this projection.

Right Anterior Oblique without Beam Angulation. In this projection, the left anterior descending coronary artery and the diagonal branches overlap, but the medial and distal portions of the LAD are well demonstrated. The proximal and midportions of the circumflex artery are foreshortened, but there is a good visualization of the obtuse marginal branches and the distal circumflex artery.

Right Anterior Oblique with Cephalad Angulation. This projection eliminates the overlapping of the diagonals and the left anterior descending coronary artery, thereby providing good demonstration of the LAD in its entire length. The proximal and midportions of the circumflex artery are foreshortened, as are the proximal segments of the marginal branches.

Right Anterior Oblique with Caudad Angulation. This projection also provides an excellent demonstration of the bifurcation of the left main coronary artery into left anterior descending and circumflex arteries. The circumflex artery is demonstrated almost in its entire length and without significant foreshortening. The origins of the obtuse marginal branches are well seen, and the marginal branches are seen in their entire length. There is, unfortunately, marked overlapping of the diagonals and the proximal and midportions of the left anterior descending coronary artery.

Left Anterior Oblique with Cephalad Angulation. Good visualization of the entire length of the left main coronary artery is obtained in this projection. The proximal segment of the left anterior descending artery is foreshortened, but there is a good demonstration of the mid and distal segments of the LAD. The origins of the intermediate diagonal arteries are well seen. The first diagonal and the proximal left anterior descending arteries overlap. The distal circumflex artery is well visualized, but the origin and proximal segments of the marginal branches are foreshortened.

Steep (60 Degree) Left Anterior Oblique. This view provides an excellent demonstration of the proximal and mid portions of the left circumflex artery and the LAD is almost its entire length.

Left Anterior Oblique with Caudad Angulation. This projection, also called the "spider view," provides an excellent demonstration of the left main coronary and the origin of both the left anterior descending and circumflex arteries.

Left Lateral Projection. In this projection, the left main coronary artery is foreshortened, but the left anterior descending coronary artery is seen in its entire length. The proximal segments of the diagonal arteries and proximal circumflex artery are foreshortened, but the mid and distal segments of the circumflex and marginal branches are well seen.

Right Coronary Artery (Figs. 13–7 and 13–8)

Using four projections, the right coronary artery can be visualized in its entirety.

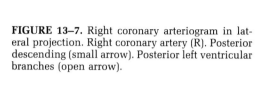
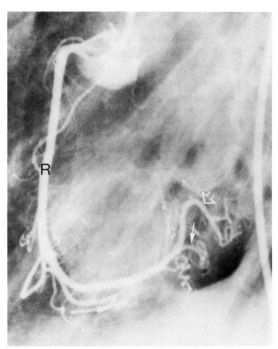

FIGURE 13–7. Right coronary arteriogram in lateral projection. Right coronary artery (R). Posterior descending (small arrow). Posterior left ventricular branches (open arrow).

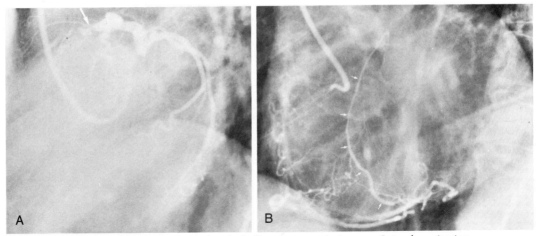

FIGURE 13–12. Coronary artery stenosis. A, Left coronary arteriogram. Lateral projection. Complete obstruction of left anterior descending coronary artery before first septal branch (arrow). B, Right coronary arteriogram. Left anterior oblique projection. Retrograde opacification of the medial and distal left anterior descending coronary artery (arrows) through collaterals.

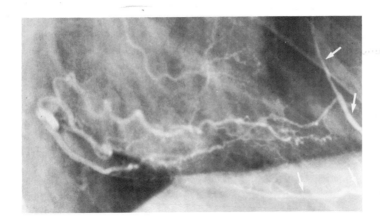

FIGURE 13–13. Coronary artery stenosis. Right coronary arteriogram. Right anterior oblique projection. Retrograde opacification of the distal and mid-left anterior descending coronary artery (arrows).

FIGURE 13–14. Nearly total occlusion of proximal right coronary artery (large arrow). Right coronary arteriogram. Extensive ipsilateral collaterals to mid and distal segments. Origin of the circumflex coronary artery from proximal right coronary (smaller arrows).

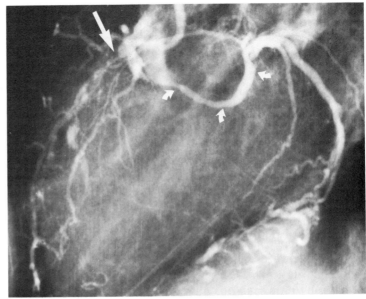

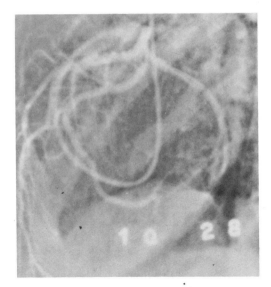

FIGURE 13–15. Common arterial trunk arising from the left coronary cusp giving origin to three major coronary vessels. Aortogram. Late phase. Lateral projection.

Studies show that coronary arteriography generally underestimates the degree of narrowing found at autopsy. The intermediate segments of the right coronary artery, the left anterior descending artery, and the proximal half of the circumflex are the segments in which underestimation most often occurs.

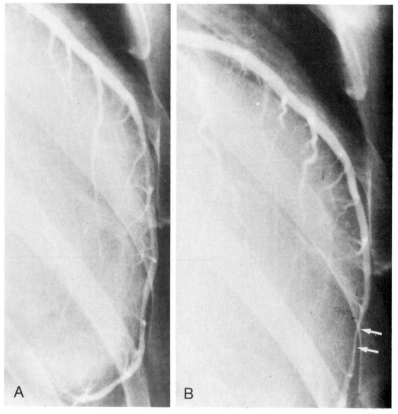

FIGURE 13–16. *A,* Left coronary arteriogram. Diastole. Normal appearance of the left anterior descending coronary artery. *B,* Systole. Area of narrowing in distal left anterior descending coronary artery (arrows).

Segments that show a uniform but relatively small vessel narrowing arteriographically may be interpreted as normal, while diffuse disease can be demonstrated pathologically in these same vessels.

Operative Management

Of the operative techniques to improve coronary blood flow, anastomosis of bypass grafts into coronary arteries beyond an obstruction (Fig. 13–17) has been the most successful. Other operative procedures, such as resection of ventricular aneurysm, closure of ruptured ventricular septal defect, and replacement of the mitral valve from mitral insufficiency, are occasionally combined with coronary artery bypass surgery. The objective of coronary bypass surgery is to produce adequate flow into coronary arteries beyond the site of obstruction, particularly under physiologic conditions of increased coronary blood flow and myocardial oxygen demands.

The results indicate that, in carefully selected cases, life expectancy is prolonged using coronary bypass surgery and that complications of coronary arteriosclerosis, namely acute myocardial infarction and sudden death, are diminished.

The incidence of acute myocardial infarction complicating bypass procedure ranges from 10 to 25 per cent, but the associated mortality is low. The operation may have the beneficial effect of alleviating angina in some cases. In other patients, the infarction may be extensive and cause severe myocardial dysfunction. In patients having extensive preoperative myocardial scarring with ventricular enlargement and poor contractility, the operation is of limited or of no value. In other instances, the arteriosclerotic disease is so extensive that adequate-sized vessels are unavailable for receipt of grafts.

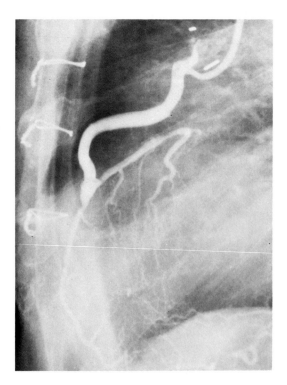

FIGURE 13–17. Injection into a venous bypass graft to the left anterior descending coronary artery. Widely patent graft and wide anastomosis. Antegrade and retrograde filling of left anterior descending coronary artery. Collateral flow through septal branches into posterior descending coronary artery.

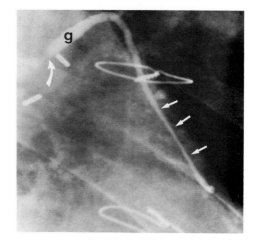

FIGURE 13–18. Injection into saphenous vein bypass graft (g) to left anterior descending coronary artery. Diffuse narrowing of medial and distal segments of graft secondary to intimal hyperplasia. Stenosis of the ostium of graft (arrows).

The bypass graft may carry an inadequate volume of blood into distal arteries, because the graft is occluded or stenosis exists in the artery beyond the anastomosis.

Occlusive changes may develop in a vascular graft. In the early postoperative period, occlusion of grafts results from thrombosis that may begin at the anastomosis and involve the entire length of the graft. Obstruction results occasionally from an inadequately sized anastomosis. Rarely, the graft twists and becomes obstructed.

Late obstruction of grafts usually results from intimal hyperplasia of the graft (Fig. 13–18). Evidence of this process is found after one postoperative month. Intimal hyperplasia may progress, and by three months the graft may be totally occluded. The disease process includes smooth muscle and fibroblasts in the tissue lining of the graft. Thrombosis may further complicate this process.

Left Ventricular Aneurysm. Left ventricular aneurysms are generally complications of myocardial infarction. Congenital left ventricular aneurysms are quite rare.

FIGURE 13–19. CT scan three days after myocardial infarction. An area of myocardium with decreased density is seen around the apicoseptal wall of the left ventricle (arrows), representing the area of the infarct. (Courtesy of M. J. Lipton, M.D., and C. B. Higgins, M.D.)

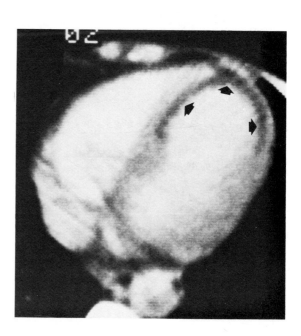

Aneurysms of the left ventricle produce localized abnormalities of left ventricular wall movement. Hypokinesis, akinesis, dyskinesis (paradoxical systolic expansion of the aneurysm), or asynchrony that represents a disturbed temporal sequence of contractions results.

There may be no abnormal radiographic findings, or there may be a localized bulge of the left ventricle, abnormal pulsation, or intramyocardial calcification.

Left ventricular aneurysms are demonstrated by radionuclide flow studies and more precisely by left ventriculography. The latter is routinely done as part of coronary arteriography. Digital subtraction angiography is a newer technique that is used to evaluate left ventricular function and to demonstrate the functional abnormalities resulting from aneurysms. Computerized tomography can provide useful information regarding the location and extent of the infarction (Fig. 13–19).

Selected Bibliography

Basu, A. K., and Gupta, D. S.: Haemodynamics in mitral stenosis before, during and after valvotomy. Br. Heart J., *24*:445, 1962.

Bjork, V. O., Lodin, H., and Malers, E.: The evaluation of the degree of mitral valve insufficiency by selective left ventricular angiocardiography. Am. Heart J., *60*:691, 1960.

Bruschke, A. V. G., Wijers, T. S., Kolsters, W., and Landmann, J.: The anatomic evolution of coronary artery disease demonstrated by coronary arteriography in 256 nonoperated patients. Circulation, *62*(3):527–536, 1981.

Chandler, A. B.: Relationship of coronary thrombosis to myocardial infarction. Mod. Concepts Cardiovasc. Dis., *44*(1):1–6, 1975.

Clark, W. S., Kulka, J. P., and Bauer, W.: Rheumatoid aortitis with aortic regurgitation. Am. J. Med., *22*:580, 1957.

Galloway, R. W., Epstein, E. J., and Coulshed, N.: Pulmonary ossific nodules in mitral valve disease. Br. Heart J., *23*:297, 1961.

Graigner, R. G.: Interstitial pulmonary oedema and its radiological diagnosis. A sign of pulmonary venous and capillary hypertension. Br. J. Radiol., *31*:201, 1958.

Jarchow, B. H., and Kincaid, O. W.: Post-stenotic dilatation of ascending aorta; Its occurrence and significance as roentgenologic sign of aortic stenosis. Proc. Staff Meet. Mayo Clin., *36*:23, 1961.

Klatte, E. C., Tampas, J. P., Campbell, A. A., and Lurie, P. R.: The roentgenographic manifestations of aortic stenosis and aortic valvular insufficiency. Am. J. Roentgenol., *88*:57, 1962.

Lavender, J. P., Doppman, J., Shawdon, H., and Steiner, R. E.: Pulmonary veins in left ventricular failure and mitral stenosis. Br. J. Radiol., *35*:293, 1962.

Melhem, R. E., Dunbar, J. D., and Booth, R. W.: The B lines of Kerley and left atrial size in mitral valve disease. Radiology, *76*:65, 1961.

Potts, J. L., et al.: Varied manifestations of left atrial myxoma and the relationship of echocardiographic patterns to tumor size. Chest, *68*:781, 1975.

Thomas, K. E., Winchell, C. P., and Varco, R. L.: Diagnostic and surgical aspects of left atrial tumors. J. Thorac. Cardiovasc. Surg., *53*(4):535–548, 1967.

Wilson, M. G., and Lim, W. N.: The natural history of rheumatic heart disease in the third, fourth, and fifth decades of life. Circulation, *16*:700, 1957.

Cardiac Tumors. Cardiac tumors are rarely primary, with atrial myxoma being the most common.

Breast and lung are the most common primary tumors metatasizing to the heart.

Increased cardiac size is the most common radiographic finding, which may be either generalized or localized. The tumor may simulate cardiac chamber enlargement. For example, a tumor of the right ventricle may mimic right ventricular enlargement, or it may cause chamber enlargement, as when a left atrial myxoma obstructs the mitral orifice, producing left atrial enlargement. In such patients, the radiographic findings resemble mitral stenosis. Pericardial effusion may occur and may be the only abnormal roentgen finding.

Selected Bibliography

Potts, J. L., et al.: Varied manifestations of left atrial myxoma and the relationship of echocardiographic patterns to tumor size. Chest, *68*:781, 1975.

Thomas, K. E., Winchell, C. P., and Varco, R. L.: Diagnostic and surgical aspects of left atrial tumors. J. Thorac. Cardiovasc. Surg., *53*(4):535–548, 1967.

AORTIC ANEURYSMS

Aneurysms are localized bulges of the aorta that may be either fusiform (involving the entire aortic circumference) or saccular (involving only a portion of the aortic circumference). The former is usually the result of atherosclerosis, the latter the result of syphilis (seen in Fig. 11–21). Patients with aneurysms often have other serious conditions such as hypertension, ischemia, or cerebrovascular disease.

Causes. The diseases causing aneurysms tend to involve specific portions of the aorta, and thus the location of an aneurysm is a clue to its cause. For example, aneurysms of the abdominal aorta are usually of atherosclerotic origin and result from atrophy and fibrous replacement of the vessel media and adventitia. Aneurysms of the descending thoracic aorta and aortic arch can be caused by either arteriosclerosis or syphilis; often, the two types can be distinguished on the basis of the extent of the circumference involved.

Syphilitic aneurysms usually affect the ascending aorta and aortic arch and are the result of inflammatory changes of the vessel with calcification and fibrosis. Often, more than one site is affected. In many of these patients, the heart, especially the aortic valve, is also affected by the disease. Cardiovascular syphilis is the result of acquired rather than congenital infection and affects principally middle-aged (35 to 50 years) men.

Marfan's syndrome causes cystic medial necrosis in the ascending aorta and leads to aneurysms. It is associated with marked dilatation of the aortic sinuses. Often, intimal tears develop and may result in dissection (see Fig. 8–18C).

Uncommon causes of aortic aneurysms are trauma and mycotic endocarditis involving the aorta.

Clinical Features. The clinical findings depend upon the size and location of the aneurysm, the type and extent of damage to nearby structures, and the damage done by the underlying disease. For example, many patients with arteriosclerotic abdominal aneurysms are asymptomatic, the lesion being discovered incidentally as a pulsatile mass or by radiographic examination performed for some other reason. In contrast, patients with syphilitic aneurysms often have aortic insufficiency, even left-sided failure. There may be distended neck veins and edema and cyanosis of the face, neck, and arms as a result of compression of the superior vena cava by an aneurysm in the ascending aorta. On the other hand, if the arch is involved, respiratory signs and symptoms are prominent. In older men with syphilitic aneurysms, radiographs of the buttocks may reveal radiopaque densities representing deposits of bismuth, which was once used to treat primary syphilis.

Aortic aneurysms produce no unique electrocardiographic signs.

Radiographic Features. Dilatation of the ascending aorta produces prominence of the intermediate segment of the right cardiac border in a posteroanterior projection (Fig. 13–21A). Dilatation of the aortic root in Marfan's syndrome may not be evident in a posteroanterior projection but causes retrosternal fullness in a lateral projection (Figs. 4–13A and 9–18C).

Dissecting Aneurysm

A dissecting aneurysm results from the entry of blood into the aortic media, usually through a tear in the intima. Dissection probably occurs only in an

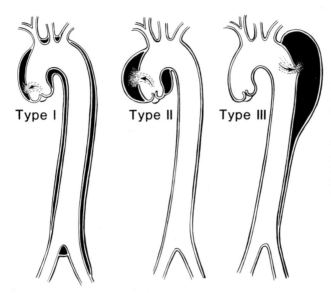

FIGURE 13–20. Types of dissecting aortic aneurysms. Type I, Dissection involves the ascending aorta and aortic arch and extends distally for varying distances; Type II, dissection is limited to the ascending aorta; Type III, dissection originates at or distal to the left subclavian artery, extending distally for varying distances. There is no involvement of the aorta proximal to the left subclavian artery.

abnormal media, such as atherosclerosis or Marfan's syndrome. The dissection usually begins in the ascending oarta either immediately above the aortic valve or immediately beyond the origin of the left subclavian artery. The blood dissects through the media and extends distally and may involve the brachiocephalic or other arteries, either dissecting along them or narrowing their orifices. The dissection may rupture into the mediastinum, pericardium, pleural space, or retroperitoneal tissues, or it may re-enter the aortic lumen.

Classification. Dissecting aneurysms have been classified by DeBakey on the basis of the site of the intimal tear and the extent of dissection (Fig. 13–20). Type I dissections are the most common, accounting for 70 per cent of the cases.

Clinical Features. Dissecting aneurysm often presents suddenly as a "cardiac catastrophe." Severe pain, often described as "tearing," may radiate to the lower back; the focus of the pain changes as the dissection progresses. Depending on which branches of the aorta are affected, there may be hemiplegia, paraplegia,

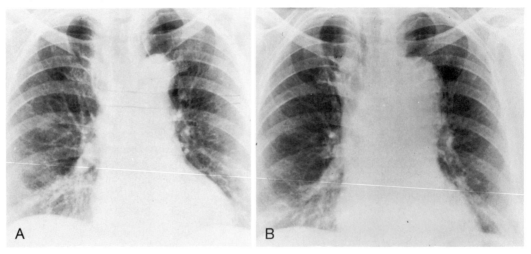

FIGURE 13–21. Aortic aneurysm. Thoracic roentgenogram. Posteroanterior projection. A, Before, and B, following dissection of aortic aneurysm. A, Normal pulmonary vascularity. Normal cardiac size. Prominent aortic knob. B, Widened upper mediastinum.

renal failure, or other signs. There may be no peripheral pulses. In severe cases, the patient is pale and sweaty, with low blood pressure; death often occurs within 48 hours. In other cases, hypertension is present.

Radiographic Features. The mediastinum is widened (Figs. 13–21 and 13–22), the aortic arch is straightened, and the surrounding structures are compressed.

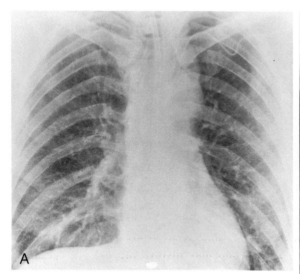

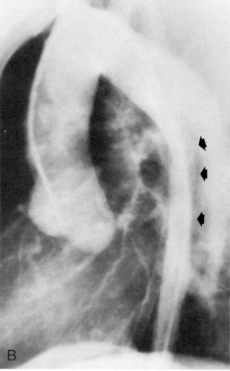

FIGURE 13–22. Patient with hypertension and chest pain. *A,* Thoracic roentgenogram. Normal pulmonary vascularity. Normal cardiac size. Widened upper mediastinum. Obliteration of the aortic knob. *B,* Aortogram in anteroposterior projection. Intimal flap (arrows) beyond the left subclavian artery. *C,* Lateral aortogram. Radiolucent band in proximal descending aorta representing an intimal flap with intimal tear beyond the origin of the left subclavian artery.

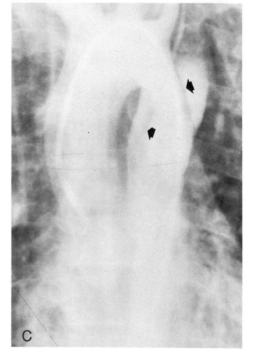

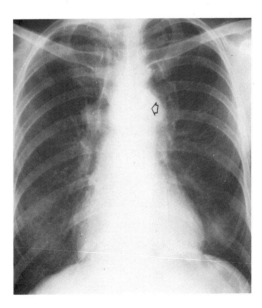

FIGURE 13–23. Dissecting aneurysm with rupture into left hemithorax. Large left pleural effusion. Wide upper mediastinum with calcification in aortic knob being medial to outer margins of mediastinum (arrow).

Ideally, an old film should be available for comparison (Fig. 13–21). A pathognomonic finding is a double aortic knob with a 1-cm separation between the outside of the aorta and its calcified intima (Fig. 13–23). Cardiomegaly may be seen if there is hemopericardium. Left ventricular hypertrophy or pleural effusion may be present (Fig. 13–23).

Angiographic Appearance. Aortography is the most accurate means of diagnosing a dissecting aneurysm and of determining its extent (Figs. 13–22B and C, 13–24 and 13–25). Recently, computed tomography (Fig. 13–26) and ultrason-

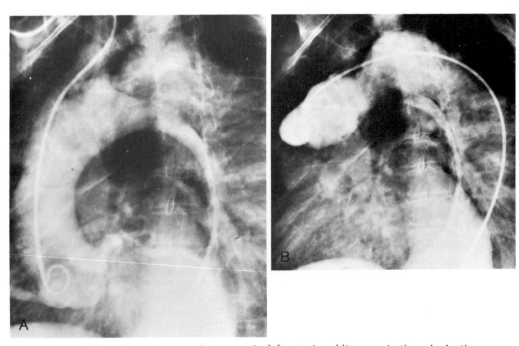

FIGURE 13–24. Dissecting aneurysm. Aortogram in left anterior oblique projection. *A,* Aortic lumen compressed at the level of the aortic arch and descending aorta. Insignificant aortic imcompetence. *B,* Injection into false aortic lumen.

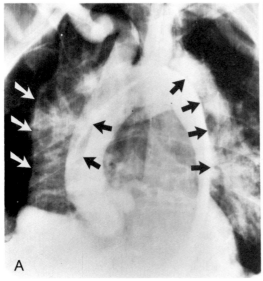

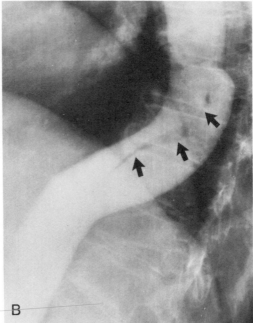

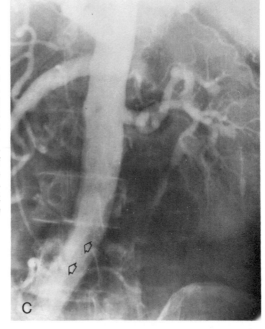

FIGURE 13–25. Dissecting aortic aneurysm. *A,* Ascending aortorgam. Anteroposterior projection. Wide upper mediastinum (white arrows). Extensive compression of lumen (black arrows) of both ascending and descending aorta by false channel filled with unopacified blood. Intimal tear occurred at level of left subclavian artery and dissected both antegrade and retrograde. *B,* Descending aortgram. Large linear filling defect within aortic lumen representing intimal flap proximal to site of reentry of false channel into aortic lumen (arrows). *C,* Abdominal aortogram. False channel extends into abdominal aorta compressing lumen (small arrows). Right renal artery and left iliac artery opacified from false channel.

ography (Fig. 13–27) have proved to be of value in the noninvasive diagnosis of dissecting aneurysm. Digital subtraction angiography can also demonstrate both the true and the false channel.

Management. Complications of aneurysms include rupture and thrombus formation with embolization. Treatment depends on the location and cause. The prognosis is poor, especially when the aortic valve and coronary and brachiocephalic arteries are involved; death within 48 hours is common, and fewer than 25 per cent of patients survive two weeks. Operative resection of the aneurysm and replacement with a graft are indicated.

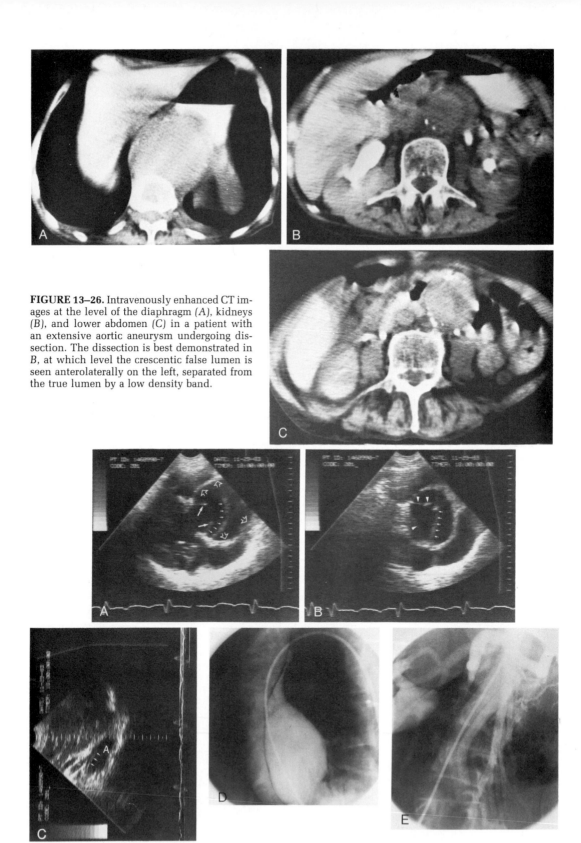

FIGURE 13–26. Intravenously enhanced CT images at the level of the diaphragm *(A)*, kidneys *(B)*, and lower abdomen *(C)* in a patient with an extensive aortic aneurysm undergoing dissection. The dissection is best demonstrated in *B*, at which level the crescentic false lumen is seen anterolaterally on the left, separated from the true lumen by a low density band.

FIGURE 13–27. Aortic aneurysm. *A,* Real time long-axis echocardiogram reveals dilatation of the aortic root (open arrows). Aortic valve leaflets in open position (large arrows) and a large intimal flap (small arrows). *B,* Short-axis reveals open aortic leaflets (arrow heads) and intimal flap (small arrows). *C,* Intimal flap is seen extending into the abdominal aorta (small arrows) at the level of the superior mesenteric artery (M). *D,* Aortogram. Dilated aortic root. Linear radiolucency in the center represents intimal flap. *E,* Abdominal aortogram. Linear radiolucency parallel to catheter represents intimal flap, which extends into the left external iliac.

Selected Bibliography

Brown, O. R., Popp, R. L. and Kloster, F. E.: Echocardiographic criteria for aortic root dissection. Am. J. Cardiol., *36*:17, 1975.
DeBakey, M. E., Henly, W. S., Cooley, D. A., et al.: Surgical management of dissecting aneurysms of the aorta. J. Thorac. Cardiovasc. Surg., *49*:130, 1965.
Dinsmore, R. E., Willerson, J. T., and Buckley, M. J.: Dissecting aneurysm of the aorta; Aortographic features affecting prognosis. Radiology, *105*:567, 1972.
Hayashi, K., Meany , T. F., Zelch, J. V., et al.: Aortographic analysis of aortic dissection. Am. J. Roentgenol., *122*:769, 1974.

Abdominal Aneurysms

Radiographic Features. Linear calcifications are commonly seen in the wall of aneurysms (Fig. 13–28). A mass effect can be produced by large aneurysms (Fig. 13–29).

Angiography demonstrates clearly the superior and inferior extension of the aneurysm. Involvement of the abdominal aorta branches by mural thrombus is well seen (Fig. 13–30).

The diagnosis of abdominal aortic aneurysm is easily and accurately established by ultrasonography, which demonstrates the extent and size of the lesion and the presence of any mural thrombus (Figs. 13–31 and 13–32). Computed tomography can also establish the diagnosis, although multiple sections are needed to demonstrate its extent (Fig. 13–33). Rupture with retroperitoneal hematoma is better demonstrated by the latter method (Fig. 13–33). Demonstration of rupture by angiography is difficult. Usually, a "nipple"-like protrusion can be seen at the site of a possible rupture. Extravasation is seldom seen.

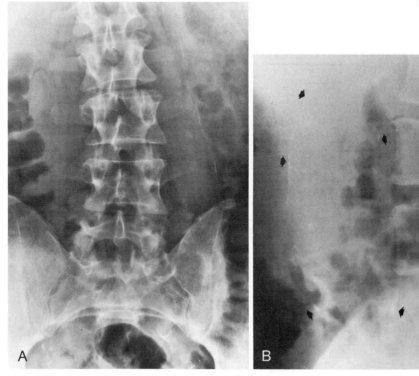

FIGURE 13–28. Abdominal aortic aneurysm. Abdominal aortogram. *A,* Flat plate of abdomen. Heavy linear calcifications adjacent to left transverse processes of lumbar spine. *B,* Lateral plate of abdomen. Extensive linear calcifications (arrows) in walls of abdominal aorta.

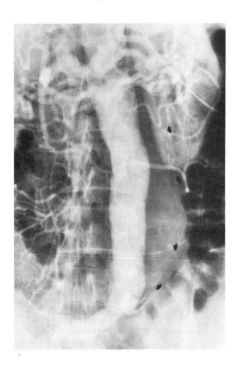

FIGURE 13–29. Large aneurysm of abdominal aorta with eccentric channel and extensive mural thrombus along left margin of aneurysm (arrows). Translumbar approach. Aneurysm extends to level of renal arteries. Lumbar arteries absent. Characteristic finding from extensive mural thrombosis occluding the ostia of these arteries.

In Marfan's syndrome there is dilatation of the aortic root with enormous enlargement of the sinuses of Valsalva. The aneurysm usually stops at the origin of the brachiocephalic vessels (see Fig. 4–13C). Dissections of the intima are a common complication (see Fig. 4–18C), and cardiomegaly is present.

Management. When atherosclerotic aneurysms reach a diameter of 7 cm, the

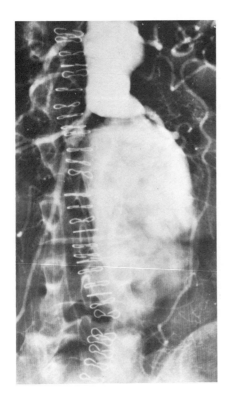

FIGURE 13–30. Abdominal aortogram. Large aneurysm of abdominal aorta below renal arteries extending to the aortic bifurcation.

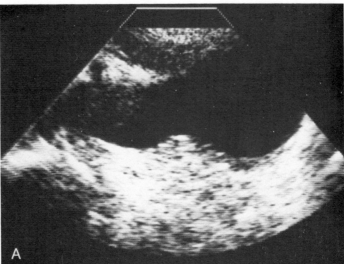

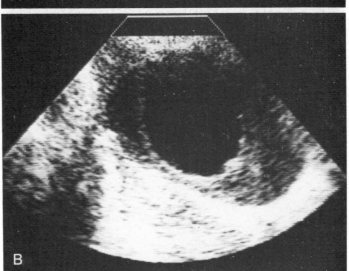

FIGURE 13–31. Longitudinal (A) and transverse (B) ultrasound images of large abdominal aortic aneurysm containing mural thrombus. Note discrepancy between external dimensions of aneurysm and dimensions of lumen.

affected segment of the aorta is usually replaced with a prosthetic graft because large aneurysms often rupture. In patients with Marfan's syndrome, the ascending aorta should be replaced when its diameter exceeds 4.5 cm. It is usually necessary to replace the aortic valve during the same operation. In contrast, an aorta involved in an active mycotic infection (Fig. 13–33) is rarely treated surgically until the organisms have been eradicated because of the potential for infection and destruction of the graft.

Traumatic Aneurysms

Deceleration injury to the aorta commonly causes rupture of the ascending aorta at this level of the isthmus.

Angiographically, the tear can be demonstrated easily. It can involve a part of or the complete circumference, with extravasation of contrast into the periaortic hematoma (Figs. 13–34 to 13–36). Dissecting aneurysms starting at the site of the intimal tear are uncommon (Fig. 13–36). If the patient survives without surgical therapy, a false aneurysm will form (Fig. 13–37).

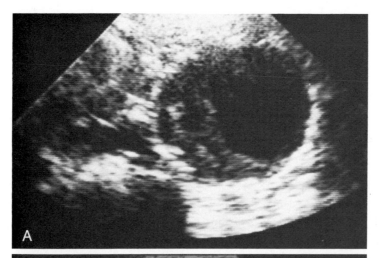

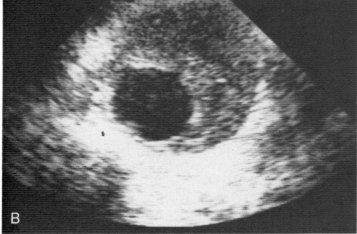

FIGURE 13–32. Transverse ultrasound images of two patients with large abdominal aortic aneurysms showing eccentricity of the aortic lumen due to mural thrombus. The mural thrombus in *A* demonstrates variable echogenicity, indicating inhomogeneous composition.

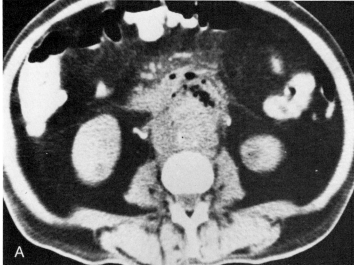

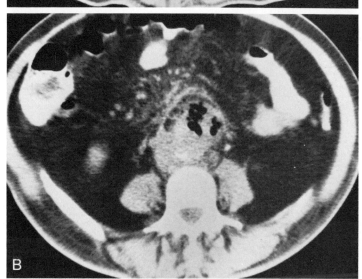

FIGURE 13–33. *A*, Ruptured mycotic abdominal aortic aneurysm. Intravenously enhanced C. T. images of distal abdominal aorta showing obliteration of the tissue planes with loss of normal aortic-caval interfaces with multiple small gas collections; *B*, lower section shows loss of retroperitoneal landmarks due to extension of gas-forming infection within and beyond a false aneurysm. Pathogenic organism: *Escherichia coli*. Surgical and bacteriologic confirmation.

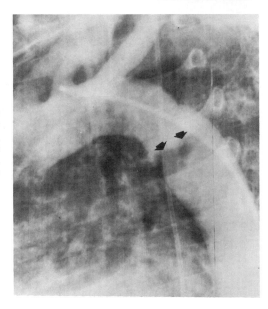

FIGURE 13–34. Traumatic aortic aneurysm with multiple rib fractures. Descending aortogram in left anterior oblique projection. Typical dehiscence of aorta distal to subclavian artery. Filling defect (arrows) represents either rolled up media or thrombus. At operation, complete dehiscence of aorta at site of thrombus demonstrated by angiograms.

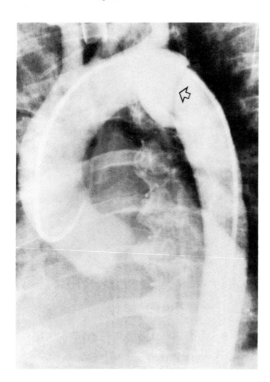

FIGURE 13–35. Traumatic aortic aneurysm. Thoracic aortogram. Extravasation of contrast medium beyond left subclavian artery. Band of radiolucency in media (arrow).

FIGURE 13–36. Traumatic aortic aneurysm with multiple rib fractures. Large tear of thoracic aorta at the isthmus with extra-arotic hematoma (H), compressing aortic lumen (A).

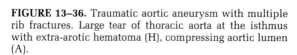

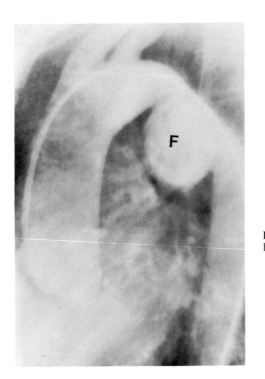

FIGURE 13–37. False aneurysm (F). Narrowing of aortic lumen at the isthmus.

Selected Bibliography

Griffin, J. F., and Koman, G. M.: Severe aortic insufficiency in Marfan's syndrome. Ann. Intern. Med., 48:174, 1958.

Pappas, E. G., Mason, D., and Denton, C.: Marfan's syndrome. A report of three patients with aneurysm of the aorta. Am. J. Med., 23:426, 1957.

Smith, W. G., and Leonard, J. C.: The radiological features of syphilitic aortic incompetence. Br. Heart J., 21:162, 1959.

PULMONARY HEART DISEASE (COR PULMONALE)

In pulmonary heart disease, hypertrophy and dilatation of the right ventricle result from disorders of pulmonary parenchyma or function. The latter may be of pulmonary or extrapulmonary origin. Right-sided heart disease secondary to left ventricular failure or to left-to-right shunts is not included in the definition or discussion.

Causes of Cor Pulmonale

The origins of cor pulmonale are often considered to be vascular and include both acute and chronic embolism or thrombosis, idiopathic pulmonary hypertension, and hypoxic pulmonary vasoconstriction. The latter category includes chronic obstructive pulmonary disease and the less common extrapulmonary conditions: central nervous system disorders causing hypoventilation; deformities of the chest such as kyphoscoliosis that interfere with mechanisms of breathing; chronic neuromuscular disease of the chest; and morbid obesity. Whatever the cause, the underlying problem in cor pulmonale is alveolar hypoxia leading to pulmonary arterial hypertension. Right ventricular systolic pressure rises, and right ventricular hypertrophy and, ultimately, failure follow.

Pulmonary Embolism and Thrombosis. Pulmonary embolism or thrombosis may develop either acutely or chronically and may be associated with a variety of conditions, including long-term immobility, rheumatic heart disease, childbirth, fractures (especially of the long bones), iatrogenic injury, and blood dyscrasias. The embolic material may be blood clots, fat (usually associated with fractures), erythrocytes (in sickle-cell anemia), air (in iatrogenic injury), or amniotic fluid. The blockage of pulmonary capillaries by the embolic material leads to hypoxia, which leads, in turn, to pulmonary hypertension.

Acute Cor Pulmonale. This condition is caused by the sudden occlusion of at least two thirds of the pulmonary circulation and is characterized by the sudden onset of pain simulating myocardial infarction, dyspnea, and shock with a disproportionate degree of tachycardia. There may be tricuspid insufficiency, with a systolic murmur and hepatic and jugular venous pulsations. Acute pulmonary hypertension is discernible by a right atrial gallop and accentuated closure sounds of the pulmonary valve.

The electrocardiogram often shows peaked P waves in leads II and III, right-axis deviation, and a characteristic S1Q3T3 QRS pattern. Complete or incomplete right bundle branch block may be noted. Abnormal Q waves are seldom found in lead II, and this helps differentiation of acute cor pulmonale from myocardial infarction.

Primary Pulmonary Hypertension. This is a rare condition with a predilection for women aged 20 to 40 years. The pulmonary arterial pressure equals or is slightly below the systemic levels. The etiology is unknown. The disease is rapidly progressive and lethal.

This rare disorder is manifested as fatigue, weakness, dyspnea, reduced effort tolerance, and congestive heart failure. Angina, effort syncope, and cyanosis may also be features. There may be a family history of a similar condition. Sudden death is a frequent outcome.

Diseases of the Tracheobronchial Tree. The major tracheobronchial diseases leading to cor pulmonale are bronchitis, asthma, and emphysema. During acute episodes of bronchitis or asthma, pulmonary hypertension is uncommon. These diseases produce emphysema, and imbalances between ventilation and perfusion develop that lead to wasted ventilation, increased dead space, intrapulmonary shunting, hypoxemia, and acidosis. If the pulmonary changes are widespread, pulmonary hypertension appears. Hypoxemia also leads to polycythemia, increased blood viscosity, and pulmonary vasoconstriction. The injured pulmonary tissue is susceptible to infection that destroys pulmonary capillaries. In response to the increased pulmonary arterial pressure, the large pulmonary arteries dilate and become atheromatous. The acidosis and hypercapnia may cause cerebral vasodilation and papilledema.

Chronic Obstructive Pulmonary Disease. The common clinical findings of chronic obstructive pulmonary disease are rapid breathing, wheezing, prolonged expiration, restricted thoracic movement, and disordered consciousness. Increased venous pressure produces hepatomegaly and distended neck veins. Heart sounds are difficult to hear because of dampening by the emphysema. A gallop rhythm and the murmur of tricuspid insufficiency may be audible in the epigastrium.

The past history of these patients usually reveals asthma, environmental or occupational exposure to pollutants, or heavy cigarette smoking. Patients have often been afflicted for some time with a productive morning cough that they accept as normal. A history of effort dyspnea may be elicited.

Electrocardiographic features include right-axis deviation, low voltage in the limb leads, clockwise rotation of the precordial leads, and, frequently, the S1, S2, S3 syndrome.

Musculoskeletal Disease. Musculoskeletal diseases reduce effectiveness of breathing and lead to inadequate ventilation and hypoxemia. Pulmonary infections are common.

Pickwickian Syndrome. This syndrome, which appears in only a small percentage of morbidly obese patients, apparently results from an insufficient sensitivity of the brain to carbon dioxide. The patients are oftne polycythemic and are subject to pulmonary emboli.

Echocardiographic Features

The anterior wall of the right ventricle is thickened, and the internal diameter is increased (Fig. 13–38). The pulmonary valve shows a diminished "a" wave and a flat E-F slope. Echocardiography is especially helpful in distinguishing primary pulmonary hypertension from hypertension associated with congenital heart disease or mitral stenosis.

Radiographic Features

Embolic Disease. Distention of the main pulmonary artery segment, cardiomegaly from right ventricular enlargement, and peripheral oligemia are common. In a few instances, abrupt termination of the vessels at the site of the occlusion may be found, but in most cases the findings are nonspecific.

Chronic Obstructive Pulmonary Disease. The radiographic findings differ, depending on the type of underlying disease. The radiographic changes of early

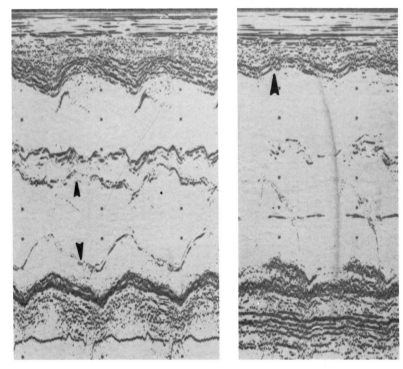

FIGURE 13–38. Pulmonary hypertension. M-Mode echocardiogram. *Left,* Flattened interventricular septal motion (arrows). *Right,* Thickened right ventricular wall (arrow).

FIGURE 13–39. Chronic obstructive pulmonary disease. Hyperinflation of both lungs with flattening of the hemidiaphragms. Large central hilar vessels, with rapid tapering toward the periphery. Normal heart size with a prominent main pulmonary artery segment.

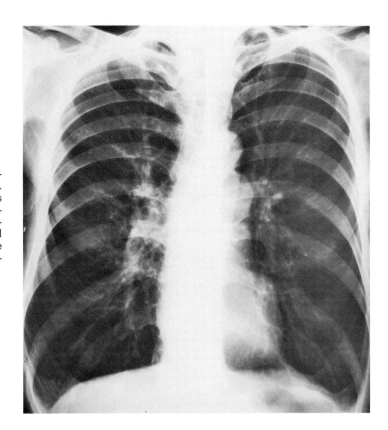

emphysema are difficult to identify. Usually, the heart is positioned more vertically than normal, the lung markings are reduced, and the hemidiaphragms are flattened. The pulmonary outflow tract and main pulmonary arteries are enlarged (Fig. 13–39). Cardiac size may be normal, enlarged, or reduced, depending on the circumstances.

Management

Pulmonary heart disease is difficult to treat effectively. Infections may be difficult to eradicate, and digitalis and diuretics have little or no effect. Efforts to improve pulmonary function usually have little or no effect. Efforts to improve pulmonary function usually fail, since the pulmonary damage has developed chronically and is irreversible.

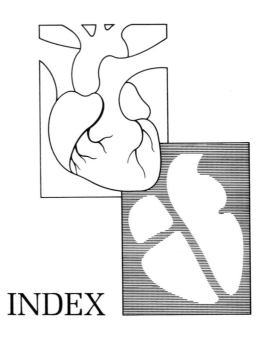

INDEX

In this index, numbers in *italic* refer to illustrations; numbers followed by (t) refer to tables.